A troupe of porcupines is milling about on a cold winter's day. To keep from freezing, they move closer together. When close enough to huddle, however, they start to poke each other with their quills. In order to stop the pain, they spread out, but again begin to shiver. This sends them back to each other, and the cycle repeats, as they struggle for a comfortable place between entanglement and freezing.

Praise for *Schopenhauer's Porcupines:*

"Deborah Anna Luepnitz has written a masterpiece about the living, breathing relationship of psychotherapist and client. A must-read for anyone engaged in psychotherapy—from either side of the relationship."

—Linda Austin, M.D., author, *What's Holding You Back?*

"Lively, graceful and moving."

—Susie Orbach, Ph.D. author of *The Impossibility of Sex*

"This is a lovely book. Few therapists are able to write as convincingly about their work as Deborah Anna Luepnitz. In describing her patients' struggles with desire, she helps us make sense of our own. Drawing on a deep reserve of psychoanalytic knowledge, *Schopenhauer's Porcupines* shows how such wisdom can change lives."

—Mark Epstein, M.D., author, *Thoughts Without a Thinker*
and *Going on Being*

"Luepnitz loves her work, writes clearly, and produces an engaging and informative book for patients, therapists and those who enjoy well-told stories."

—*Booklist*

"This truly rare collection teaches essential issues about hard-won intimacy, hate-in-love, and the connection between the psychic and the social. Here post-Freudian theory descends from its couch into the streets. Luepnitz's formidable charm comes from her ability to take us along as she strolls like a witty, keen-eyed Lacanian, full of insight and compassion."

—Jean-Michel Rabaté, Ph.D., author of *The Future of Theory*

"In this age of quick-fix cures and Prozac-for-tots, I'm glad to have a book to give to those who ask: "But how can *talking* help?"

—Thelma Jean Goodrich, Ph.D., *Families, Systems, and Health*

"Deborah Anna Luepnitz offers us a challenge: to reconsider the role of dialogue in the therapeutic encounter, which lately has focused far more on pharmacology. In these finely wrought tales, the reader comes to see for the first time, or comes to remember as if from a long time ago, how two people may speak their way into a new kind of sense, and, by doing so, widen the world."

—Lauren Slater, Ph.D., author, *Welcome to My Country* and
Lying: A Metaphorical Memoir

"Of all the social myths that govern our lives, that of 'true love' may be the most intractable. *Schopenhauer's Porcupines* helps us understand how we fall into romantic traps and how talking therapy can be liberating in the deepest sense. A splendid achievement."

—Nancy Hollander, Ph.D., psychoanalyst and author of
Love in a Time of Hate

"Beautifully crafted, free of jargon, this is a remarkable account of what really happens in therapy. Luepnitz does more than tell gripping stories from her professional past: she also rediscovers that past anew on the page. The results—literary and psychological—are impressive."

—Andrew Samuels, author, *Politics on the Couch*

Also by Deborah Anna Luepnitz

THE FAMILY INTERPRETED

SCHOPENHAUER'S

DEBORAH ANNA LUEPNITZ, Ph.D.

PORCUPINES

Intimacy and Its Dilemmas

FIVE STORIES OF PSYCHOTHERAPY

BASIC
BOOKS

A Member of the Perseus Books Group

Designed by Lovedog Studio

Library of Congress Cataloging-in-Publication Data
Luepnitz, Deborah Anna.
    Schopenhauer's porcupines : intimacy and its dilemmas : five stories of
psychotherapy / Deborah Anna Luepnitz
        p.   cm.
    Includes bibliographical references (p.).
    ISBN 0-465-04286-4 (hc); ISBN 0-465-04287-2 (pbk.)
    1. Psychodynamic psychotherapy—Case studies. 2. Transference (Psychology)—Case
studies. 3. Resistance (Psychoanalysis)—Case studies. 4. Psychotherapist and
patient—Case studies. 5. Luepnitz, Deborah Anna. I. Title.

RC489.P72 L84 2002
616.89'14—dc21   2001043499

03 04 05/ 10 9 8 7 6 5 4 3 2

FOR GRACE

The only victory in love is escape.

—Napoleon

... [T]he God of woman is autonomy.

—Alice Walker

be of love(a little)
More careful
Than of everything

—E. E. Cummings

CONTENTS

MAKING ROOM IN LOVE
FOR HATE

> He said his little statues and images helped
> stabilize the evanescent idea, or keep it from
> escaping altogether.
>
> H.D., *Tribute to Freud*[1]

IT IS A CLEAR London morning, unusually bright for November, and I am making my way to number 20 Maresfield Gardens. I have visited the Freud House many times, but today will be different: the museum's director has offered me time behind the velvet ropes.

It is a common fantasy, I suppose, to walk alone through the great art collections of the world. The objects in these particular rooms shaped Freud's reflections on the unconscious, making the visit particularly poignant for the likes of me, a psychoanalytic psychotherapist.

Erica Davies is a Welsh woman with cornflower-blue eyes and a detailed knowledge of the two thousand or so objects in the house. She dates a number of pieces for me: Greek, Etruscan, Coptic, Roman. Where, I ask, is the statue of Athena

---

[1]Notes—both bibliographic and explanatory—appear at the end of the book (see p. 250). Henceforth, numeric callouts will not appear.

mentioned by the American poet Hilda Doolittle in the exuberant memoir of her analysis with Freud?

"She is *here*."

Erica taps the small sculpture with a respect that is familiar, almost casual. The gods are used to her.

"And what can you tell me about this porcupine?" I point to a bronze figure, its back to the ancients, crouched in the middle of the desk.

My guide smiles. More is known about the ancient Egyptian *shabtis!* The porcupine was a gift to Freud from psychologist G. Stanley Hall on the occasion of Freud's only visit to America in 1909. According to one account, Freud claimed he was going to America to catch sight of a wild porcupine *and* to give some lectures. This whimsical remark apparently was meant to deflect anxiety about lecturing. But why a porcupine? We know only that the founder of psychoanalysis kept the little creature on his desk and in plain view.

I ask if the statue could refer to the porcupines in Arthur Schopenhauer's well-known fable, a story Freud liked enough to cite in his book on group psychology. Erica seems delighted by my question. As we sit together over tea, I paraphrase the fable as follows:

A troop of porcupines is milling about on a cold winter's day. In order to keep from freezing, the animals move closer together. Just as they are close enough to huddle, however, they start to poke each other with their quills. In order to stop the pain, they spread out, lose the advantage of commingling, and again begin to shiver. This sends them back in search of each other, and the cycle repeats as they struggle to find a comfortable distance between entanglement and freezing.

The story spoke to Freud as a lesson about boundaries. ("No one can tolerate a too intimate approach to his neighbor.") It spoke also to his belief that love is everywhere a thorny affair. Freud wrote: "The evidence of psychoanalysis shows that almost every intimate emotional relation between two people which lasts for some time—marriage, friendship, the relations between parents and children—contains a sediment of feelings of aversion and hostility, which only escapes perception as a result of repression." Freud believed that the one exception to this was the love of a mother for her son, which was "based on narcissism," proving only that he was, among many other things, an Old World Patriarch.

In the 1940s and 1950s, British pediatrician and psychoanalyst Donald Winnicott elaborated on the subject of love/hate relations between parents and children. In a classic paper, he listed some eighteen reasons why the ordinary, loving mother might hate her infant—daughter *or* son. (For example: The baby endangers her body during pregnancy and delivery. He may be cranky and implacable all morning, and then go out and "smile at a stranger.") Winnicott maintained that mothers who could acknowledge the discomfiting fact that love—even for babies—is ambivalent would be less likely to do harm than the disavowers. Winnicott, I think, would have enjoyed the observation made by novelist Fay Weldon: "The greatest advantage of not having children must be that you can go on believing you are a nice person. Once you have children, you understand how wars start."

All relationships, not just familial ones, require us to contain contradictory feelings for the same person. As the poet Molly Peacock has observed: "There must be room in love for hate."

Definitions of love, aggression, intimacy, and privacy vary enormously, of course—by culture, historical moment, and social class. Without making universal claims, we can assume that people in the contemporary West, with the possible exception of cloistered nuns, live lives bedeviled by the porcupine dilemma. That is, we struggle on a daily basis to balance privacy and community, concern for self and others, sexual union and a room of our own.

•   •   •

One year after I wrote the above, a young woman applicant to a cloistered religious order was sent to me for psychological evaluation. She seemed genuinely ascetic and contemplative, and I said so in my report. Her spiritual advisor was not as cheered by this as I expected. These young women, she said, will spend the rest of their lives relating only to each other, and thus require exceptional social skills. A Carmelite cloister, I learned, is no place for a loner. Porcupines are we all.

Although we know these dilemmas to be commonplace, we don't always experience them as such. For example, an affable thirty-five-year-old divorcee, a lawyer, who had grown up with loving, adoptive parents, sought my help for depression. She enjoyed her work and her friends but was chronically unhappy in her intimate relationships. Moreover, like many women in their mid-thirties, she experienced loneliness as a personal failure rather than as a condition quintessentially human.

"There may be something really wrong with me," she said in tones befitting one who robs orphanages for sport. "When there is no man in my life, I feel empty and unlovable, and can barely enjoy anything. When I get close to a man, I feel smothered and pampered, sort of chubby with love. I long for time to think, to work late, to feel the edges of things, just to be. Is this sick or what?" A number of things went through my mind, having to do with her earliest attachments, her childhood fantasies about adoption, and her actual experiences with men. For some reason, perhaps because she was so keen to call herself bad names, I decided to tell her the fable of the porcupines. I will never forget her response:

"It's *soothing.*"

Others have said the same. The fable normalizes a problem that many of us take for nothing less than a bizarre character flaw.

There is a more familiar story about love and connection, also cited by Freud in passing. It comes from Plato's famous dialogue the *Symposium.* In that dialogue, Socrates and friends gather to dine and to discuss the question: "What is love?" The response that most readers remember is the one given not by Socrates but by Aristophanes. Aristophanes explains that in the beginning of time people did not exist in single bodies as we do now but, rather, were pairs joined at the shoulder. There were three types of pairs: male-female, male-male, and female-female. These twin-type creatures tumbled around all day, carefree and, of course, never lonely. One day they did something to offend Zeus, who cut them in half as punishment. Afterward, they walked around lonely indeed, searching endlessly for their other half. And so it is to this day, declaimed Aristophanes, that human beings wander through life looking for the person who will complete them, for in our true and original nature, we were not one but two.

Whether or not we have read the *Symposium* or heard the story elsewhere, most of us were weaned on the idea of what we might call Aristophanic love. Modern culture and, indeed, whole industries depend on people's obsession with perfecting themselves in anticipation of finding their ideal mate. During that moment in our lives when we feel this kind of love, if we

ever do, stories about making one out of two please us enormously. However, when we are alone, or with someone who
does not make us feel whole, our culture's romantic myths
serve up heaps of reproach.

Moreover, in view of evidence all around us that no perfect
complements exist, the lure of romantic merger endures, while
the prospect of solitude terrifies. For many single people in the
West, it is the dreaded, deadly alternative to happiness. For
those who enjoy it, solitude is a guilty pleasure. For still others,
solitude is a state devoutly to be wished, something unattain-
able because of the demands of work and family. This may account in part for westerners' interest in various Eastern
philosophies. Countless Americans have dabbled in Buddhism,
studied yoga, or learned to meditate, in search of a quiet mind.

Arthur Schopenhauer (1788–1860) believed he understood
something important about human desire and its dilemmas. He
saw unhappiness as inexorably part of our design. The existence of what he termed "will" was a permanent source of discomfort, meaning that there simply is no life without suffering.
Schopenhauer's notion of will was not a matter of personal
agency—"what I want"—but almost the opposite: a blind
striving that characterizes all living things. Its most insistent expression in human beings, he said, was sexuality. Writing *contra*
the eighteenth-century myth of "rational man," Schopenhauer
argued that reason was forever in conflict with the will, and
that the latter was more commanding than most of us acknowledged. Thus, for Schopenhauer, our only real chance at
contentment lay in the eradicating or transcending of the will.
Saints and geniuses might do this for a lifetime. The rest of us
could escape the thrum of appetite periodically through aesthetic experience. When absorbed in art, literature, or music, he
said, we free ourselves from the prison of will.

If the notion of "life as suffering" sounds suspiciously Hindu, it is. Schopenhauer was the first Western philosopher to study the Vedic and Buddhist texts. Their influence shines through his (initially ignored) *The World as Will and Representation*, and also through his later popular essays and aphorisms.

The *Upanishads* were helpful to him in his personal life as well. Schopenhauer, by all accounts, was a repulsive man who preferred the company of dogs to people. He was ill-tempered and once pushed a neighbor down a flight of stairs for disturbing him. Living in relative isolation, he warmed himself by the fires of philosophy and the pleasures of art. Permitted a moment of psychologizing, we might guess that his educated and wealthy parents, in their own ways, schooled his pessimism. The father, an anxious, exacting man, committed suicide when his son was seventeen. And Arthur quarreled with his mother, who threw him out and never saw him again after he was twenty-six. Whether his relationship with her was the cause or effect of his misogyny is hard to determine. We do know that he was prone to depression and wrote: "I always have an anxious concern that causes me to see and look for dangers where none exist." He referred to the sacred Hindu texts as "the consolation of my life."

. . .

Schopenhauer interests me because of his place in the history of psychoanalysis. It was he (in advance of Freud) who broke with the Enlightenment view of the self as rational and unified. He anticipated not only the Freudian unconscious and fascination with sexuality but also the significance of slips of the tongue and the interpretation of dreams.

The crucial difference between Schopenhauer and Freud is that the latter invented a clinical method—psychoanalysis—to address the suffering born of our divided nature. Ever since the patient known as "Anna O." coined the term "talking cure," countless women and men the world over have engaged in psychoanalysis and the scores of therapies it has spawned, including Gestalt, marital, group, and family therapy.

It would be difficult to overestimate the impact of psychoanalysis on Western minds. Freud has left his mark on philosophy, religion, education, law, art, literature, film making, even jazz. Benjamin Spock, whose *Baby and Child Care* has sold more copies than any other book in history except the Bible, acknowledged "Freudian psychoanalysis" as the "underlying psychology" of his work. In 1939, W. H. Auden could claim without hyperbole that Freud's name referred no longer to a man but to "a whole climate of opinion."

America's attitudes toward the talking cure nonetheless remain ambivalent. It is true that many people in the public eye have "come out" as psychotherapy patients with the intention of removing the stigma. As early as 1956, in fact, *ur*-comedian Sid Caesar appeared on the cover of *Look* magazine, describing within its pages his own salutary years on the couch. More recently, activists, intellectuals, and popular artists—including Gloria Steinem, bell hooks, Cybill Shepherd, and Carlos Santana—have mentioned publicly their experience with talking therapy. There can be little doubt, however, that significant social stigma remains. An elected official can lie to the public and survive, but to lie down on an analyst's couch would mean political death. This taboo reflects the American ethic of self-reliance. It is driven by our love affair with medicine and the attendant belief in the magic of pills. Roughly one in ten Americans have taken Prozac or one of the other selective serotonin reuptake inhibitors (SSRIs). Physicians have prescribed these drugs for half a million children, despite disturbing data on long-term use.

How to explain this apparent triumph of medication over talk? Gaps in public awareness may be more responsible than cost. Drug companies spend billions educating (and misinforming) consumers about the potential benefits of their products. What most Americans know about therapy, however, comes from television shows and movies that depict therapists as benign bunglers, sexual predators, or competent folks who just can't say no to helping mobsters. Some of these representations are hilarious (*Deconstructing Harry*) and well-written (*The Sopranos*); others, simply banal (*The Prince of Tides, Good Will Hunting*). It is strange but true that people still come to therapy not knowing what to expect, and asking the same question: "How can talking help?" It was a question I myself asked as a young woman entering therapy for the first time.

Many practitioners believe that talking therapies provide a "corrective emotional experience." Such therapies, they maintain, offer the abused or neglected person an experience of respect and recognition—a new psychic reality. Some researchers have argued more recently that psychotherapy alters our brain chemistry along the lines of the serotonin-elevating medications. But whatever their merits, theories alone can't describe the connection between "talk" and "cure." This is achieved best through case stories—those written by therapists or patients.

The first such book written for a lay audience, Robert Lindner's 1954 *The Fifty-Minute Hour*, remains one of the best. The paperback cover reads: "I am a psychoanalyst. I meet and work with murderers, sadists, sex perverts—people at the edge of violence—and some who have passed that edge. These are their stories as they told them to me—searching, revealing, perhaps shocking."

If Lindner's rhetoric is overheated and his therapeutic persona a bit heroic, the treatment he describes is intelligent and effective. He worked hard to dispel the notion (still rampant) that psychoanalytic therapy is only for rich neurotics. Engaged and compassionate with patients, he also dispatched the myth of the supercilious analyst, distracted and prone to dozing off in session.

Among the psychoanalytic case books published in the decades following, Susie Orbach's *The Impossibility of Sex* may be the finest. Writing from the perspective of a feminist relational psychoanalysis, Orbach explores the use of the countertransference—the psychological and even physical responses of analyst to patient—with exceptional rigor. Orbach's cases, like those of many other therapist authors, are fictional. In creating "patients-on-the page" she solved the problems of disguise and confidentiality, but faced other difficulties. Certain readers, apparently, cannot help but object: "This therapy seems compelling, but if you tell me you made up the cases, then how do I know it really works?"

There is no perfect solution to the problem of writing about therapy patients. But not to do so strikes me as the riskiest choice at a time in our culture when the power to define madness, malingering, and suicide potential is being handed over to insurance company functionaries.

My imperfect solution has been to write stories about real (but carefully disguised) patients who have graciously granted me permission to do so. I have tried to render faithfully the substance of the clinical work, while changing information that could identify actual people. I also offered patients the chance to choose their own disguise, including pseudonyms.

My purpose here is no more nor less than to add to the legacy of Lindner, Orbach, and others who have given lay readers the opportunity to learn what goes on inside the consulting room. There are no "murderers or sex perverts" here, nor anyone suffering from odd neurological disorders—no one mistaking wife for hat. The patients I describe are people living through garden-variety marital despair, sexual misadventures, medical terrors, and creative impasses. They are white, black, mixed race, straight, and gay. One was wealthy, one poor, the others working and middle class.

During the treatment, which ranged in length from a few months to fourteen years, neither they nor I knew that I would one day write about them. This is a question best raised only after treatment is done, so as not to unduly shape it.

Over the course of twenty-five years, I have had patients who were not satisfied with what I had to offer, and who left what I would call "prematurely." (They may have called it "not a minute too soon.") Those people are not represented here. Indeed, patients unhappy with their therapist are unlikely to give such permission.

Readers may ask if altering identifying material does not make case histories fictional. In *My Life as a Man*, Philip Roth's Peter Tarnapol, a novelist and a Jew, upbraids his analyst, Dr. Otto Spielvogel, for disguising him in a professional article as an Italian-American poet. Tarnapol describes as "dim-witted" the assumption that ethnicities are interchangeable. Regarding the switch in vocations, he fulminates: "And while we're on it, Dr. Spielvogel, a poet and a novelist have about as much in common as a jockey and a diesel driver."

I am sympathetic with that argument, and dislike having to alter biographical facts for the sake of confidentiality. (How does one disguise a patient's experience of being struck by lightning?) At the same time, we know that illness mocks the distinctions of place and fortune. The depressions of the novelist, poet, and truck driver can be depressingly similar.

My project, in any case, is not biographical. The main character of these stories is not the patient but the process—the

talking cure. I have tried to describe the week-to-week unfold-
ing of therapy—the setting of fees and the interpretation of
dreams, the exhilarating detective work and the inevitable te-
dium, the wrong roads taken and the occasional thrill of arrival. Conveying these facets of therapy remained more
pressing than actual demographics, events, and faces.

The cases presented here are not examples of classical psychoanalysis. The first case describes a married couple in treatment, and the second a family. The individual patients were not
lying down on the couch four to five times a week but sitting
up once or twice weekly. What defines psychotherapy as psychoanalytic (as opposed to behavioral or cognitive) is the attention given to unconscious processes and especially *transference*
and *resistance*. Freud wrote: "Any line of investigation which
recognizes these facts [transference and resistance] and takes
them as the starting point of its work has a right to call itself
psychoanalysis, even though it arrives at results other than my
own." The concept of transference turns on the fact that we
don't meet other people as much as we construct them, based
on previous experiences going back to childhood. Freud observed that we are especially apt to construct the analyst or
therapist in the image of our parents. The same therapist will
be experienced by one patient as a forbidding father and by another as a compassionate mother. Consider a prospective patient who, after three preliminary sessions, wrote me a letter
saying she had decided to start therapy with me. The letter,
which held high praise for my warmth and insight, took a
month to reach me because the patient had used a California—
not a Pennsylvania—zip code. It was, moreover, not just any
California zip code, but her mother's—a woman she had described as critical and cold. The transference relationship had
already begun. That is: while the patient sincerely believed me

to be different from her mother, her unconscious had conflated us. On recognizing the mistake, the patient said that she had indeed worried that after officially becoming my patient, once she was my "captive audience" I would treat her differently, critically.

People can spend a lifetime experiencing the world as the cruel (or withholding or indulgent) parents of childhood. Psychotherapy provides the opportunity to take notice of these assumptions and call them into question. The transference includes all the feelings, thoughts, fantasies, and actions evoked in the patient in contact with the therapist. And the countertransference is the set of feelings, thoughts, fantasies, and actions evoked in the therapist in contact with the patient.

Freud believed that the countertransference was a problem—perhaps a sign that the analyst needed more analysis. An important contribution of the British school was reformulating the countertransference as something both ineradicable and useful to the treatment—a source of information about the therapeutic process itself. If I notice that I'm feeling disconnected from (or bored with, or protective toward) a patient, I ask myself why I might be feeling that way at that particular moment in the treatment. These feelings are never to be enacted, and only rarely disclosed to the patient. But if they go unnoticed by the therapist, they can derail the treatment.

The example of the wrong zip code also touches on the issue of resistance—sometimes defined as the setting up of obstacles to the treatment. Resistance is not a bad thing; it is something not to be crushed but to be respected and understood. As much as we come to therapy in the hopes of changing, so do we also want to remain the same. Our neurotic symptoms—painful and vexing as they can be—are familiar. They also talk for us when we are unable to find words. The patient used the wrong zip code, perhaps, because she was afraid of saying, "I've got your number!" The mistake had the result of slowing things down for this young woman who was indeed nervous about beginning treatment.

Psychoanalytic therapists differ enormously in their style, which in turn varies from patient to patient. With some people, I find myself talkative; with others, more abstemious. The late French analyst Serge Leclaire said it best when he remarked that "Psychoanalysis must be re-invented for each patient."

Many groundbreaking clinicians and theoreticians have influenced my work. I will be citing Freud throughout, and also Winnicott, Lacan, and a number of psychoanalytic feminists. Donald Winnicott is best known for his concept of the "transitional object," which makes its first appearance in our lives as the security blanket of childhood and later includes music, art, and all forms of creative endeavor. If Freud saw the goal of analysis as enabling people "to love and to work," Winnicott seemed to add a third essential element: love, work, and *play*. From him I have learned the importance of creating a "holding environment" for the patient—an atmosphere of safety and trust like the one mothers provide for babies. Only in such a space will patients take the risk of revealing more than a false or compliant self.

It was also Winnicott who coined the controversial term "good-enough mother." Certainly it has been misused by his followers in ways that implicate mothers in everything that can go wrong in a human life. Winnicott's definition of the good-enough mother, however, was nonsentimental. She is "one capable of having a straightforward love-hate relationship with her infant."

Jacques Lacan, the iconoclastic French analyst and philosopher, is bound to be less familiar to English-speaking readers.

Unlike Winnicott, Lacan wrote in a style that is extravagantly difficult even for other analysts. Throughout his career, Lacan remained critical of what he saw as other analysts' attempts to make patients conform to bourgeois social codes. He believed, for example, that the emphasis on mother-baby love in the work of British analysts eclipsed attention to adult sexuality and the erotic in general. If Winnicott's key word was "mothering," Lacan's was "desire." For Lacan, desire is what simultaneously defines us as human subjects and what prevents us from ever being whole or complete. To desire something, after all, is to lack something. Whereas Winnicott's tropes tended toward the organic—he spoke of "growth," "development," and "maturity"—Lacan's imagery was more somber. ("The cipher of his mortal destiny" is characteristically Lacanian.) For Winnicott, only in illness was the self divided, while for Lacan human subjectivity was necessarily divided, because of the existence of the unconscious. No matter how successful we become, no matter how much we are loved, we will always be vulnerable to irrational fears and capable of the most self-defeating acts. As Freud said, we can never be "master of our own house."

The family was important to Lacan, but his conception of its influence went well beyond the nuclear unit. Decades before family therapists were talking about "the intergenerational transmission of psychopathology," Lacan was insisting that analysts needed to understand three (not just two) generations in order to comprehend an individual's symptom.

One of Lacan's most famous teachings is expressed in his enigmatic statement "The sexual relationship does not exist." Lacan didn't mean that people don't fall in love or revel in sexual pleasure. He meant that the sexual relationship for which most of us yearn—the ideal, Aristophanic type in which divided

human beings are made whole—does not exist. From the Lacanian perspective, we might say that the romantic story from
the *Symposium* corresponds to the Winnicottian worldview, which
begins with a blissful mother-baby union. For Lacan, there never
was perfect union with the mother, so the romantic "refinding"
of her (for both sexes) can only be imperfectly gratifying. Only
those who know themselves as *lacking* are even capable of love,
according to Lacan.

The integration of Winnicott and Lacan into one master
theory would be impossible. Their works are divergent, and in
some ways incompatible. Lacan, for example, insisted that the
goals of analysis were not "therapeutic." For him, psychoanalysis involves allowing the subject of the unconscious to
speak. Patients often feel better and live better as a result, but
the analyst must be careful not to step out of position by educating or comforting the patient. Winnicott had no contempt
for therapy. He practiced both psychotherapy and psychoanalysis, depending on the needs of the patient, and was not
against offering comfort. He hoped to promote "an alive experiencing" that would foster the patient's ability to love and
communicate in intimate relationships. Lacan was less interested in promoting communication than in helping people
reckon with the thing most suppressed in Western societies—
the fact of our mortality.

Devotees of the British and French traditions have been
known to point their pens at one another and say, in effect,
"What *we* do is psychoanalysis, and what *you* do is not."

Having learned a great deal from both Winnicott and Lacan,
I have come to think of them as representing, respectively, the
comic and tragic values in the rich tableau of psychoanalytic
thought. Comedies end in marriage; tragedies, in death. (Think
of the plays of Shakespeare, for example.) In Winnicott we

find a benign worldview and an ameliorism—a belief that health and happy families are possible, and that humankind can change for the better. In Lacan we are more apt to encounter a Freudian pessimism—a sense that there is something fundamentally unmanageable about human existence, making words like "health" extremely suspect. If collapsing these views into each other would be futile, disregarding one or the other seems almost phobic.

Twenty-first-century practitioners may be better off working inside these theories' vast and exhilarating contradictions. I will let the case examples speak to the success and failure of my efforts to do just that.

•   •   •

To return to my earlier question: How does talking help?

A twenty-five-year-old music teacher sought treatment for panic attacks so disabling that he could not keep a steady job or sustain a relationship. He hesitated to seek help because he thought a therapist would blame his "normal, hard-working" parents for his misery. He saw his family infrequently, and always paid a price in increased panic attacks for days after a visit.

He had been close to his sister as a child, but now he found her company repellent. They disagreed on politics and religion and often hung up on each other after a brief spat. My patient urged me not to make a big deal about this. All his friends said the same thing about families: You avoid them like the plague until some combination of guilt and dependency sends you home. "Come on," he replied, irritated by my questions. "These weren't violent, mentally ill child molesters. They were hard-working parents who did their best."

One year of talking complicated this simple picture. My patient would not have characterized his father as "violent," he said, because he had never hit the kids, and punched his mother on only three occasions that he knew about. Although his mother was depressed, he would not have called her "ill." Her habit of driving drunk while the kids cried for her to stop could be explained. She felt ignored by her husband, and this was her only way of getting his attention. At the age of ten, my patient was paid by a male relative for sexual favors. He could not have told either parent, of course, because "it was important for me to keep my parents calm."

Didn't all families have problems? he asked. Didn't all kids worry about these things?

Far too many children call emotionally and physically destructive places home, but this doesn't make those homes normal in the sense of benign. Unlike the lawyer mentioned earlier, whose problems with intimacy were fairly typical but who experienced them as odd and shameful, this young man had learned to normalize pathology.

What talking therapy helps us do is to separate the particular catastrophes of our family and social circumstances from the general catastrophe of having been born human and, thus, subject to aging, death, and the dilemmas of intimacy caricatured in Schopenhauer's fable.

As a result of speaking first to me and then to his sister, the teacher's life changed. The two of them stopped competing and finally cried together about their frightening early years. Together they approached their adult cousins about the abuser, who was now babysitting for the younger generation. Eventually, the members of this family were able to develop a much more straightforward love-hate relationship with each other.

The young man's panic attacks stopped within a year, and he began the first passionate sexual relationship of his life.

In this kind of work, the stakes are astronomically high. The ways we love or abuse our intimates—the ways we allow ourselves to be loved and abused—are passed on unconsciously. To work with one family or even one individual can stop a cycle of miseries—or at least diminish their force—for generations.

Psychotherapy cannot make us whole, but it does allow us to transform suffering into speech and, ultimately, to learn to live with desire. As these cases show, it can help turn egregious neurotic misery into the porcupine dilemmas of everyday life.

1

SAME BED, DIFFERENT DREAMS

In her 1972 classic, *The Future of Marriage*, sociologist Jessie Bernard wrote that every marriage is really two: the husband's and the wife's.

A Chinese aphorism puts it another way: "Same bed, different dreams."

.   .   .

The message on my answering machine made me sad. It was from a couple I had treated three years earlier, a husband and wife who seemed to be doing well enough when we said good-bye. I recognized the light Greek accent as Daphne's:

"Karl and I are in the middle of a crisis. We spent Friday night in the emergency room. I can't take this. I want a divorce. Please call. . . . "

When I phoned back, they were out. I left a message, then sat down to think about them.

The emergency room?

They had no history of violence. Neither one had ever mentioned suicide. Their initial request had actually been for family therapy, involving Melina, Daphne's then-thirty-year-old sister, who lived with them.

I remembered the first time I went to greet them in the waiting room of the training hospital where I was working at the time. One receptionist whispered to another, "That new guy over there looks like Fabio."

Her colleague replied, "The wife could be Cher." I had no trouble spotting them. Karl Loeb, a forty-year-old construction worker, had a blond ponytail, tar-black eyes, and a long, thin nose. His muscular build was the kind that made chairs look too small for him. Karl's beefy hand circled the wrist of Daphne, a lissome thirty-six-year-old with smoldering brown eyes and long hair set off by rhinestone earrings. One might have expected languorous gestures from someone so lovely, but Daphne was restive and tense. At that moment, she was styling her sister's hair with quick, birdlike movements. A sweet-looking redhead, Melina was resisting the uninvited make-over with one hand while putting on her glasses with the other. She was the first to meet my gaze.

This image of them stayed with me like a snapshot of the family structure. Karl couldn't get close enough to his wife, who had eyes mainly for Melina, who was definitely in the picture but wanted Daphne out of her hair.

Walking over to them, I remember feeling pleased and confident. At thirty-two, with five years' experience seeing patients, I still had a lot to learn. But fewer new patients were looking me over and asking, "How long have you been doing this, dear?" I introduced myself and invited them back to my office.

The problem this little family brought to me was that they were making each other miserable. After Melina's husband walked out on her and their three-year-old daughter, Lily, she had asked to move in with her sister and brother-in-law "for just a few months." The few months had become four years, as Melina struggled to pull her life together. Then their mother died, drawing the sisters closer still.

Daphne was energetic, well-organized, and neat. Melina was an easy-going person who could tolerate a mess. Daphne hectored her daily about showing some drive. Melina would then attack Daphne for being "up my nose all the time," but she also invited interference by regularly running out of gas, money, and babysitters. Karl had long been the peacemaker, but he was getting tired of it. The battle had reached its current pitch three weeks earlier when Daphne learned she was pregnant. She had married late, and was thrilled finally to be having her own child. She wanted things settled before her baby was born.

As easily as those early sessions could become shouting matches, it was clear that there was a great deal of love in their household and that the fighting between the sisters masked a dense loyalty. Although they insisted that living together had become intolerable, even the most tentative question from me about Melina moving out set them both to weeping.

In time, all three came to realize how they had unconsciously arranged the current situation to distract them from the pain of the mother's death from breast cancer. Melina had suffered two major losses in four years, and was acting childlike to ward off the apprehensions of living alone. And as much as Daphne wanted her space back, she had loved having her niece there. Seven-year-old Lily brought a daily joy that helped mitigate the memory of the mother's excruciating illness and death. Daphne had to mourn the fact that her mother would never know the child she was carrying. Motherhood was the one thing that would have made her a success in the eyes of her parents, now both deceased.

The sisters recognized that they were duplicating a drama from the previous generation, as their mother and her sister had stayed bonded together with "super glue." The metaphor was Daphne's: "They were glued together with that stuff that tears your skin off if you're not careful."

What had passed from one generation to the next was a habit of loving that some therapists call "enmeshment." Mourning freed them up and made them ready for change. Over the course of five months of sessions, the three adults, and especially the sisters, began to feel the kind of genuine closeness that autonomy alone permits.

Was it their goal to continue to live as a family? It was not. Melina landed a good job and moved out. She also took her ex-husband to court for child support.

When Melina visited each week, the sisters were glad to see each other. What impressed me most was that Daphne had been able to say to Melina the words "I miss you" and, later, "I love you." Ironically, many people who are enmeshed in each other's lives are not able to say those things. For them, there is no space between the "I" and the "you" for "love" to fit.

After Melina and Lily moved out, Daphne found herself unhappy with Karl. For all the squabbling between the sisters, Melina had been a good companion, more emotionally present than Karl. If Daphne needed to talk over a decision about the holidays, or an altercation with a neighbor, Melina was there, easy to engage. Karl was not a big talker; his idea of a supportive moment was rubbing her neck as he watched whatever game was on the sports channel. If Daphne read something in the newspaper that incensed her, Karl would tell her to relax: World hunger was not her fault. As for housework, it was easier to do his share than hear him grunt at her reminders. She felt she was living with an adolescent boy, and she longed for adult company.

With just the two of them in the house now, and the baby due in just a few months, Daphne asked Karl to remain in therapy so they could work on their relationship.

Karl said he wouldn't mind, but he considered their marriage "near perfect." Daphne, in contrast, felt her list of grievances mounting. *He* felt they were temperamental opposites who complemented each other. She felt overworked and underloved. They were a case in point for Jessie Bernard's dictum: "Every marriage is really two." Daphne's was an unhappy marriage, and Karl's was fine—except for Daphne's unhappiness.

The problems they were having just a month after Melina left were not unlike those of the two sisters. Daphne saw Karl as lazy. Construction work was seasonal, and he should be doing everything to line up other jobs, now that they had a baby coming. Daphne was also bothered by the fact that his main interest was wrestling. She wanted to spend weekends at the orchestra or ballet. The fact that he did not want—in her words—"to better himself" put her in a dither. Both came from working-class, immigrant families, and both had lived at home until they were adults. She had managed to finish two years of college, working long hours and living frugally to save for a house. Karl, in contrast, was profligate. He had been introduced to gambling in his twenties, and gambling became his life for a ten-year period he described as "harrowing." He had reached the point of borrowing from loan sharks to pay off gambling debts. He would then borrow more money to place bets. He was the youngest of five children, tolerated by a blustering German father and adored by a beleaguered Polish mother. She, at times, would lend him money for gambling.

When Karl first met Daphne, he was dazzled by her good looks. He overheard her telling off a co-worker and decided she was "part Greek goddess, part street tough." The combination suited him.

Daphne loved his kindness and his sense of humor, and was not aware of the gambling.

"It's not your average stereotype, is it—a blond construction worker who gambles? But gamblers come in all shapes and sizes," she said. "There are some women, too." Daphne said she was drawn to Karl's handsome face. She seemed reticent to acknowledge that their extremely satisfying sexual relationship was one of her main reasons for marrying him. She actually asked me if that sounded like an awful thing to say.

The question caught me off guard, and I tossed out: "Why? Wonderful sex is important—especially to keep a marriage going."

Daphne looked at me as though I had just revealed secrets for splitting the atom. She repeated my simple words quietly, with obvious relief. A more experienced therapist would have explored this area further: Why did she feel it was an awful thing to say? With whom did she associate that idea? Fortunately, she was able to make use of my bluff remark.

Sex had continued to be the only uncontested area of their relationship. At this point, all other issues—chores, leisure, work, and English grammar—were combustible.

Karl and Daphne had not completely lost sight of the good they had done each other. Purveyors of extremes, they knew they had pulled each other toward some emotional center. Daphne had become less compulsive; Karl had moved from dissolute to responsible.

As a condition for marriage, Daphne insisted that he get help for the gambling. She did her research and found out about Gamblers Anonymous (GA), a twelve-step program modeled after AA. He agreed to attend meetings and decided to follow the program. That meant abstention from gambling of all kinds. GA also recommended that the gambler carry no credit cards for a while and never walk around with more than ten dollars in cash. For married members, the plan specified that their spouses handle the couple's money: the bills, taxes, purchases, and so on. It was a drastic change, but Karl was willing to follow through.

Daphne was only too happy to take on this responsibility, as it ensured that the family's money would be well-managed. And so it came about that for nearly ten years—through the buying of a house, the purchase of several cars, and four years of helping to raise their niece—Daphne had taken care of all the finances, held the credit cards, and given Karl his "allowance."

Like all the strategies we use to make relationships function, this one worked until it didn't. Daphne began to complain that handling the finances alone had become onerous. In money matters, she felt as if she was the mother and he, her son.

Talking helped. They said they had done more listening to each other in those additional sixteen weeks of therapy than in all their previous married life. By the time we stopped, three things had occurred:

1. Karl announced he was ready to handle money again, and took over the bill paying and tax figuring.
2. Daphne vowed to stop correcting him in public.
3. They agreed to alternate nights out and nights at home watching television.

The couple stopped therapy after four months because they felt they were ready to go out and "do it." The baby would be born any day, and they would have their hands full. Two weeks later, they sent me a birth announcement with a photo of a gorgeous baby named Rose—born eight months after they had set foot in my office.

·　　·　　·

As I sat waiting for them to call back that Saturday afternoon three years later, I wondered if I had agreed too soon to their ending therapy. Had Karl gotten his hands on their pension fund and gambled it away? Had Daphne clocked him in sheer frustration?

And what about the decision that Melina and her daughter move out? A colleague of mine once worked with a couple whose parents were gallingly overinvolved with them. They had even joined the newlyweds on their honeymoon. After two years of marriage, and with the blessing of their therapist, the wife announced they were taking a vacation—alone. That very night, her mother had a heart attack and died. The more I thought about the possibilities, the worse I felt.

Around dinner time I received a call from the emergency-room doctor. Daphne had been the identified patient. Her symptoms were chest pain, tachycardia, nausea, and a feeling she was about to die. The diagnosis: severe panic attack.

·　　·　　·

I have never had a panic attack, but I have treated many people who suffer from these terrifying surges of anxiety. Some believe they are dying of heart failure, and indeed, cardiac trouble needs to be ruled out. Others speak of an overwhelming feeling of dread that something terrible has happened or is about to happen. It becomes dangerous to distract oneself from the thought, even if one can, because one will remember it momentarily and feel the wave of fear again. One young woman compared the physical sensation to "breathing through the eye of a needle."

When Daphne phoned me that evening, she was already feeling better. Still ruminating over the possibilities, I was feeling worse.

This kind of exchange of emotions—one person feels better as another comes to feel worse—is a subtle example of "projective identification," a construct that will show up frequently in these cases. It involves the splitting off of one's painful emotions and, in a sense, "storing" them in another person who in some way agrees to contain them. It's not a conscious strategy for making someone else feel bad but, rather, an unconscious means of transmitting unbearable information. One could say that they delayed phoning me back because they needed me to understand their experience, to feel some inexplicable or at least unexplained dread.

Daphne had no idea what precipitated her panic attack the previous evening, but she said that two months earlier, a strange kind of fear had come over her. It would strike once a day and she would need to lie down until it passed. But yesterday had been the worst of it, for she thought surely it was her heart. When the medical tests turned out negative, and the emergency-room doctor suggested anti-anxiety medication, Daphne became angry. She said she had a therapist and wanted to speak with her immediately. She signed a release so that the doctor could share information with me.

Daphne had never before been the officially designated "patient." She boasted of never having set foot in a hospital until her baby was born. During our family sessions, she had registered

Melina as the patient, who often behaved accordingly. Similarly, in the couple's therapy that had followed, she insisted that the person out of control was Karl.

For Daphne to have a crisis was something unheard of. In session the next morning, she spoke of how hard it had been to convince Karl she was in trouble.

"He thought I was exaggerating," she said.

"I hoped she was," Karl explained. "She is the Rock of Gibraltar that everyone leans on."

Daphne had never complained of anxiety during our earlier work. She was a busy person. If she had what she called "nervous energy," she would clean a closet or strip a floor. I asked if she could remember when the first attack had occurred. She had been feeling upset since early fall, she said, when her mother-in-law had suffered a mild stroke. Though sad and anxious, she hadn't felt panicked. The first attack came only two months ago, after her daughter's third birthday party. She had been packing up Rosie's old baby clothes for a pregnant neighbor. She suddenly realized that her daughter, while hardly grown up, was no longer a baby. She spoke like a big girl and was amazingly self-sufficient. Just then Daphne had felt a wave of nausea pass over her.

"I was thinking that night about her growing up and leaving home, and I got so upset, I had to lie down."

So she did know something about the meaning of the anxiety attacks?

"Yes, I do. I know he wants to rob me of the one fulfilling thing in my life. And I have decided he won't. I will *have* another child."

This was the first I was hearing about her interest in having more children. "Insistence on" would be more accurate. And Karl, I gathered, was just as insistent on stopping at one. I asked to hear from him.

"Call me immature or lazy or what have you," he said. "I was never sure I could handle a kid of my own. I didn't think I was cut out for it. I fell in love with a woman who wanted one, so of course I wanted to have Rosie, and she is the greatest thing that ever happened to me. I felt OK helping to raise my niece, too. But now I'm forty-four, and she's forty. I want to send Rosie to college. My mother is frail, and she depends on us financially. So I can't see having more. I told her this, and this is when it hit the fan."

To me, he sounded warm and vulnerable and responsible—all the things she wanted him to be. I asked Daphne what she was thinking at the moment.

"That I wish I had married someone else, that's what! Why is he talking about college when she's three? She doesn't have to go to Harvard, you know. What are you now, a Yuppie? Is money all you think of? What about the joy of bringing new life into this world? I am not finished with this part of my life, and no one is going to tell me I am!"

I couldn't help noticing that I felt more sympathetic with Karl's point of view. In the past, my sympathies were evenly divided between them.

At the end of the session, absolutely nothing had been resolved, but they planned to return the following week.

Daphne opened the session, saying:

"For weeks I have been obsessed with the idea of having another baby. There is not one minute of the day when I'm not thinking about it. I have to do it; it almost doesn't matter how. Today I feel a *little* less obsessed. But I am still determined to get pregnant again."

Something had changed. Daphne could now state calmly that Karl needed to agree to another child—or she would leave him.

I was relieved to hear her use the word "obsessed." It suggested that she knew there was something excessive in her demand. Nearly everyone has been obsessed with a desire for something or someone at one point in time. The discomfort of obsessive thoughts has brought many a person into therapy. The session temporarily replaces the obsession. Therapist and patient work together to interpret the repetitive thoughts in question, for obsessions are rarely about their ostensible object. An obsession with germs or food usually turns out to be not about good health but about the desire to seize control and the terror of losing it. The man obsessed with his wife's attraction to another man turns out to be more fascinated with his rival than with her. The woman in love, obsessed with one self-absorbed artist after another, is actually enthralled with the creative process itself, not infrequently her own. Daphne had to know that there was something suspect, something decidedly nonmaternal, about insisting that her husband impregnate her *now* or get out of her way. If the obsession was standing in for something else, what might it be?

She had dropped several clues—too many, in fact, to pursue in a short period of time. For example, the obsessive thoughts began shortly after her mother-in-law's stroke. Had that event awakened the pain of her mother's death? Was Daphne flooded with intimations of her own mortality? If so, then the obsession with another baby might be a way of warding off fear of her own physical vulnerability, waning fertility, aging, and death. Another patient of mine had once spoken candidly of having a second baby "as a replacement child," recognizing that the one child she already had could die.

If obsessions are not what they appear to be, their decoding must take place on the patient's timetable, not the therapist's. Daphne made it clear that she did not want her obsession toyed with or examined at the moment. She wanted it taken at face value.

By the time of this second session, Karl was showing more distress than before. Picking at the seam of his jeans, he choked up as he said there was just no way he could agree to more kids.

"I can't do it. This is not like buying a new sofa, Daphne. It's some serious stuff you're talking about."

"With or without you, Karl, I am going to do it. Do you think it would be so difficult for me to find a man who would have sex with me?"

"What am I—*nothing?* I'm supposed to sit here and listen to this crap about you finding some idiot to mess around with?"

"You are not 'nothing.' You are the only man I love and have ever been with. You are making *yourself* into nothing."

"She says she can't give in on this issue," Karl fumed, looking at me. "Well, guess what? I can't either!"

Sensing we had hit an impasse, I asked about other aspects of their lives. Apart from the baby issue, things were going well. For the three and one-half years since we had said good-bye, Karl had remained in charge of the money, responsibly so. Daphne, for her part, had managed to cede control, and took pleasure in the new arrangement. They were saving money, and she had been able to stay home with Rosie, which meant a lot to her. When Daphne was a child, her mother had waitressed in a Greek restaurant and always came home spent. Daphne loved being a mom. It was something she did well. She was not finished having babies, and no one was going to tell her she was.

I remembered her saying that it was while packing up baby clothes for a pregnant neighbor that she had felt the first panic attack. Was it something about this neighbor? Did the situation evoke some particularly fierce sibling competition? Melina, her seven-years-younger sister, had been pregnant long before Daphne. We had touched on their mutual jealousy in the first round of therapy. Daphne said it didn't seem particularly relevant to what she was feeling now.

What Daphne could describe very clearly was the painful and impinging emptiness that had overtaken her for months. One thought kept recurring: If she had no baby, her life would be over. The end of pregnancy and childbirth meant a loss too awful to face, "like giving up an arm or a leg." In a few years, she observed, Rosie would be in school, and each year, her daughter would need her less. Who would she be, if not a mother?

Karl picked up on this question. He said he loved being a parent, but he also enjoyed getting out of the house each day. He didn't mind the physical labor most of the time, and his coworkers were good guys. He got pleasure from passing a completed building and saying, "I was part of that." He believed Daphne was extremely intelligent, and felt that if she could pour herself into work, she might give up the baby obsession.

I could see Daphne's movements constrict as he spoke. She did not meet my gaze, fixing her eyes instead on her cuticles, which she pushed back, one by one, as she listed the awful jobs she had held in her life. "Kennel assistant. I was bitten twice the first week. Secretary. You were told when you could pee. Short-order cook. The eighty-year-old owner would grab my thighs while I was pouring hot grease. . . . Am I making my point to the two of you? Can you not see that it was a blessing to quit work and take care of my mother, and now my daughter?"

I certainly could.

Recalling her refrain about "bettering herself," I asked if she had any interest in returning to college.

Karl lit up when he heard my question. We had reached the end of the hour, and I asked Daphne if she wanted to say anything before we finished. She looked pensive and said slowly, still looking away: "Yes, I think that is an option, of course. Education."

Two days later, there was a message from Daphne. She had decided to stop therapy, as I was obviously on Karl's side. It was not a job or a degree she wanted. She wanted another child. She had hoped that I, as a therapist and as a woman, would understand this. She was not about to pay someone to preach to her for an hour about going back to school.

I was nonplussed. We spoke on the phone later that day, and I apologized for being insensitive. It took quite a while for me to convince her that I was not trying to push her into some awful job where she would be exploited. I had wanted to help her interpret in the fullest possible terms her yearnings to produce, to create. I had not meant to imply that she should not become a mother again. Daphne accepted my apology, but that was not the end of it. She phoned again midweek saying she just could not return to therapy after what I had said. Again, I heard her out, and encouraged her to come to the session and bring with her all her anger and disappointment. Daphne was someone who had often been angry with her parents, but she had never been able to show it. It was a sign of her faith in me that she was "letting me have it" on the phone.

Daphne and Karl kept their appointment. Both looked exhausted and, indeed, had slept little during the week because of the fighting. Now the problem had spread.

"Before it was just the baby issue. Now she's creating a stink about lights left on, one dish left in the sink. We're both hoarse from screaming. Maybe she's right and we should split up. The tension is going to kill us both."

Daphne looked solemn and defeated. "Yes," she said. "Maybe this is it."

Karl added that they had argued throughout their courtship and marriage; they were both hot-blooded. In fact, he added, a lot of their arguments gave way to some of their best sex. They had often joked about this. But this was something different, these shouts and recriminations. They did not lead to amorous reconciliation. They had not had sex for five weeks—a light-year for them.

Rosie had heard them arguing one night and began crying in her room. One evening, she climbed out of her bed and stumbled downstairs, sobbing, "Don't fight, Mommy and Daddy!" They were mortified. Karl struck out at Daphne. "You're no help hollering at her for messing her diaper! She's upset already! Let her alone!"

"Leave her alone? If I don't train that child she'll be pooping in her pants until sixth grade—like you!"

"Daphne, you are sick. I'm talking about our baby freaking-the-hell-out at night, and all you can do is dump on *me*. Do you give a shit about your daughter right now?"

"How dare you question my love for my child! I am a better parent than you, and a better mother than any of your sisters. Where the hell do you get off questioning my love for Rosie?"

"I wasn't questioning your love. I was talking about first things first. Why is your main goal always getting me in a headlock? I am sick of this crap! I am sick of it, Daphne. Do you hear me?"

Their voices, superimposed, were booming. I thought I saw the lights flicker.

"You're sick? *You're* sick of this? Who is the one who got us into therapy? You had a perfect marriage, right?"

"Don't scream in here, goddamn it!"

"I am not screaming!!! We need to solve the problem of what Rosie has been doing this week. Were you going to sweep that one under the rug?"

They had always managed to keep their child out of their arguments, something few raging couples can do. Again, something had changed.

I interrupted the shouting to ask what they were referring to. At three and a half, Rosie was still not potty-trained, despite several bursts of effort on their part. What alarmed me was the news that in the past week, the child had been reaching into her diaper after a bowel movement to smear feces on the walls.

This sign of distress in their child was sobering, powerful enough to create détente. They were devoted to Rosie, and wanted to help her.

They shouted for another fifteen minutes—mostly about who was responsible for the shouting. My ears hurt. I said I had a suggestion.

"Do not suggest I get my tubes tied!"

"No, I certainly wasn't going to—"

"Do not suggest that I practice birth control of any kind!"

My suggestion was simply this: that the question of having more children be set aside for a while. We had some work to do before returning to it. If their daughter was smearing feces, something was wrong. Perhaps she was trying to create a stink of her own to stop the fighting. A new baby would enter the world at a disadvantage if the family was in an uproar. They were not to discuss the issue in therapy or at home. There was to be, in short, a moratorium on the "b" word.

Daphne said, "It's OK with me. I honestly can't take much more of this fighting. I need some normalcy and so does he, don't you?"

"Yeah, a moratorio, or whatever. I'm getting an ulcer." Near the end of the hour, Daphne asked sheepishly if I was angry with her for calling midweek to tell me off. I replied by reminding her of our discussions, three years earlier, about the taboo on showing emotions in her family of origin. In Daphne's words at the time: "My mother made us feel like, 'You're just lucky I'm here—don't rock the boat.'" The therapy boat is made for rocking.

"I didn't hurt your feelings?" she said, refusing to budge until I reassured her.

"She's been on pins and needles," said Karl. "She was saying, 'Now look what I've done. I've alienated the one person in this world who really understood me.' I said, 'Gee, thanks, Daph. Why don't you worry about alienating *me*?'"

"'When you try one-tenth as hard as Deborah has, that's when I'll worry,'" she had replied. Daphne was relieved that she hadn't damaged our relationship. Here we were doing important work in the transference. At a conscious level, Daphne wanted very much to trust my capacity to withstand her anger without getting my feelings hurt. Nonetheless, insofar as she transferred onto me the image of her mother, her trust remained shaky. I apparently chose a reasonably good moment to make an interpretation along these lines, because Daphne showed less anxiety about losing me thereafter. Obviously, she invested me with enormous powers of insight and compassion. This was not a bad thing, but my hope was that she would show Karl how to understand her ten times better.

In any case, it was a very odd session. Odd for *me*, I mean. A moratorium on the word "baby"? This was strange stuff, given that the fundamental rule of psychoanalysis is to say everything that comes to mind, no matter how pleasant or unpleasant. Was I saying I was unable to withstand the crashing surf of emotion in the room? Maybe they *needed* to scream some more. I needed to think about my countertransference. Although I wasn't yet a seasoned practitioner, I was not easily overstimulated by patients' fighting. I was not Miles, the self-described "Super-WASP" in our group of interns. Miles had never heard his parents argue and, because he had not been allowed much television, had never really heard adults raise their voices until he was in college. As a therapist, he was at home with tippling suburbanites who carried on stealthy affairs, but screaming husbands and wives made him queasy. I always thought that two weeks with my family of origin would have cured him. I grew up around noise. Overlapping voices, open rage, adult themes: Television had nothing on my family's everyday dramas. Too much passive aggression might curl my neurons, but fighting was something I usually took in stride. What was I doing, then, telling these two people to put a lid on it?

Consciously, it simply felt right to create a space for reflection. Thinking, even listening, had become difficult because of the level of emotion and the sheer din. And Rosie needed our attention.

Unconsciously, what was at stake for me? In declaring this moratorium, was I trying to quiet my own parents, or acting out the common childhood fantasy of blocking the arrival of a sibling? Perhaps. Daphne had hoped "that as a therapist and as a woman" I would understand her yearning for another baby. Two children did not strike me as excessive, certainly. My own grandmother had twelve, and my aunt had thirteen. I knew something about the price they paid, and thus nothing was more important to me as a young woman than education and having choices. Were my personal priorities preventing me from honoring the hopes of my patient? These are questions every therapist should be asking all the time, and I did indeed bring them to my own analysis and clinical supervision. As for the value of the intervention itself—the "moratorium"—that could be assessed only later, in view of the results.

Just seven days later, Karl and Daphne looked much brighter. They had done some talking during the week, and

realized they were overworked and needed some time alone together. They hadn't taken a vacation in years. During that week,
they searched out inexpensive getaways to Florida, booking
one for the spring, several months hence. Having that to look
forward to raised their spirits, and they spent the session discussing Rosie. She had not done any smearing that week, but
she was extremely clingy, refusing to let Mommy out of her
sight for a second. A friend had mentioned to Daphne that a
few hours of preschool per week was good for kids. It would
give Rosie, an only child, a chance to make friends. Daphne
liked the idea, and so did Karl.

Several sessions passed in this way, with the two of them
problem solving. They were working on the friendship aspect
of their marriage, and they were clearly enjoying each other.

The moratorium had been in effect for one month when,
near the end of a session, Daphne's face again clouded over
with displeasure. She clipped her hair on top of her head and
peeled off her vest like someone paring down for a fight.

"Karl and I were saying last night that our sessions have been
easy and nice, and it's true. But in a way I have to say, 'So what?'
We know we can get along if we avoid the thing that divides us.
That issue is not going to go away. What is the point of solving
other problems if we make no progress on the main issue?"

"She thinks we're just stalling."

"I am going to have another child, with or without him.
And I don't have forever, you know. I am already forty. How
will we know when we're ready to talk about it again? What
will be the signs?"

"She is using the 'c' word, instead of the 'b' word."

He could always make her grin.

"Really, Deborah. How will we know? I can postpone thinking about this for a while. I can't postpone it for too long,

though; the biological clock is ticking. I don't mean to be arguing with you all the time, but I think this has to be addressed."

"Speaking of the biological clock," said Karl, "our time is up for today. For now, we're back to the mora-TAR-ium, ain't we?"

"That word is pronounced *mora-TOR-ium*. And yes, I am willing to not talk about it for another week, but I think we should talk next time about how we'll know when we're ready to discuss it again. Karl, what do you think?"

"Yeah. I hate to say it, but yeah, we gotta face the music."

The suggestion gave me pause. I wasn't sure in that moment how to frame an endpoint to the moratorium. However, it was clear that they both wanted to move forward. The week flew, and it seemed like no time had passed before the receptionist rang my office to say, "The Loebs are here to see you, Dr. Luepnitz."

As soon as I sat down across from them I realized something: I had dreamed about them the night before. I could remember nothing about the dream, only that they had made an appearance. The thought made me smile. Clearly, they were on my mind. A former therapy teacher of mine named Carl Whittaker occasionally recounted his own dreams to his patients to nudge them out of an emotional rut. Reporting dreams to patients is not my style, however. It can blur the line between therapy and friendship. I said nothing.

Daphne started the session by saying that although she dreaded getting back to the main agenda, "That's why we came here."

Karl said, "I've been hoping all week one of us would get the flu so we could cancel the session. But if we don't talk about the real problem, we're wasting time and money."

I said, "On the one hand, if you talk about having another child, emotions run high and you end up in a deadlock. On the other hand, working on anything else feels a bit irrelevant. And although the moratorium gave some relief, the question is when to end it, when to jump back into that frightening dilemma. That's the question."

They nodded. Several minutes passed.

I had no solution. I decided just to rephrase the conundrum in order to clarify things, or maybe just to buy time. I continued:

"How is it possible to discuss something that can't be talked about?"

"How to get to first base without both of us screaming our lungs out?" said Karl, digging his knuckles into the back of his neck.

I had no idea where this was going.

"I guess you'll say we never really stop thinking about it," Karl continued. "It's always in the back of our minds, bubbling around the subconscious, right?"

"I hope that's true," Daphne chimed in. "Like we're working on it even when we don't know it. Is that the theory behind the moratorium? Boy, I'd love to know what you're thinking right now!" Daphne turned to me.

A quiet moment passed, and I spoke, not fully sure of what I was about to say.

"I was thinking about dreams," I said. "I agree with both of you; important questions like these never leave our minds completely. I'm thinking that it's time to pay close attention to dreams."

There are many theories about the origins and meaning of dreams. I subscribe to the Freudian view that a dream is a fulfillment of some wish. The dream tells the wish in disguise. Usually, therapists work with dreams as they arise in the course of the therapy; dreaming is not given as an assignment.

Nonetheless, it seemed that in this situation, attention to dreams might give us the best of two worlds. We could set ourselves to facing, and not avoiding, the tough question they had brought to therapy, and in a way that would be less contentious than the campaigns of recent months.

Daphne sat up in her chair.

"You can count on me. I love thinking about my dreams. I just don't know about him. You don't really dream, do you?"

"Even asleep she has to be better than me."

I mentioned that with a bit of effort—that is, by trying in the morning to remember one's dreams or writing them down—almost everyone is able to do this work.

At our next session, Karl said he had two dreams one night, but couldn't remember them in the morning. Still, he was happy to have awakened in the middle of the night knowing he had dreamed. This was a start.

Daphne told her dream:

I am at a dentist's office and find out I need two root canals. I had been eating a sandwich. The hygienist says, "It's a good thing it happened here, or you would have swallowed the filling." They pulled it out of my mouth, and I wondered.

She asked if it was all right to tell me her interpretation:

"There is a void in my life, and I want it filled. I'm glad I'm here in your office."

I had many questions and interpretive thoughts of my own about Daphne's dream, but chose not to voice them. Dream interpretation in couple's and family therapy does not always take the form it does in individual therapy. Working on dreams with more than one patient in the room is something I learned not from books or seminars but from a family in crisis years ago. I was sitting with the family of fifteen-year-old Leroy Johnson, who had been committed to our psychiatric hospital after numerous juvenile offenses. After making significant progress, Leroy had relapsed, leaving his parents angry and hopeless. We sat silently in session, no one wanting to start. I myself had tried everything with them and, absolutely out of ideas, was beginning to think that therapy was a lost cause. Leroy broke a long silence by saying he had had a dream the previous night. I invited him to recount it, and he and his parents spent the entire hour interpreting the dream. Not surprisingly, the dream went to the heart of things: Leroy's fiercely guarded longings for his biological father who had abused him and his mother. The dream offered us an indirect, less volatile way to talk about loss, grief, and violence. It cleared a space for thinking.

That session took place in the mid-1980s, and I have been working with dreams in couples and families ever since. Were Daphne working with me in individual therapy, I would have asked her to tell me her associations to each element of the dream. I would have said, for example, "Tell me about the dentist's office, about root canals, about *two* root canals, about the hygienist, about the sandwich," and so on. This could have led us in any number of directions, all pertaining to Daphne as an individual and to the nature of her transference to me. I may or may not have pointed out that the hygienist/therapist in the dream could be a mother figure. For indeed, the "void" that created the panic happened just after her mother-in-law's stroke. This surely re-evoked grief over her own mother's death. Perhaps Daphne's desire was for mothering. In caring for babies, she might enjoy vicariously the pleasures of being mothered. In couple's therapy, the focus is slightly different. I will ask both partners for associations, but it is their interaction with regard to the dream that is crucial. It is more important to ensure that the couple become accustomed to exchanging "dream ideas," using these to advance their dialogue, than to do a "complete" interpretation.

After Daphne reported her dream, she was eager to drop it and move on. Their agenda for the evening was full. They wanted me to know that they had been at loggerheads all week. Karl had called her a "dictator." She was so busy telling him what to eat and how to eat it, what to say and how to pronounce it, that even when she was clearly right about something, he could not stand to admit it. Rosie's toilet training, for example.

Daphne asked my advice on this issue, because he was driving her crazy. Together they had decided that it would be best for Rosie to join a playgroup a few hours a week. The school's requirement, however, was that children be toilet trained.

Karl said he wanted Rosie trained, but that it was "torturing her" to use the potty. The routine in the house was as follows. Daphne would put Rosie on the potty and read to her. She would cajole and encourage and sometimes leave the bathroom for a few minutes, knowing that this often led to results. If Karl was in the vicinity, however, Rosie would start to cry, and he would rush in and take her off the potty. "He is teaching her that if she screams, she will get her way," Daphne argued.

Karl replied, "It does make me the good guy. But I think Daphne is wrong to let her cry."

Daphne volunteered the information that Karl had not been trained until the age of five.

"It's true. I remember it. My father would scream about 'that filthy little shit-ass,' and my mother would defend me and say I was just a baby. Before kindergarten, she made sure I was trained."

"Karl was her youngest. She smothered him. It was almost sick."

"Maybe my mother didn't read Dr. Spock, but I turned out OK. Now Daphne, here, was toilet-trained from birth. So she is Mrs. Clean, and won't let anyone forget it. So who is sick, I ask you?"

Experts on eating disorders at the Women's Therapy Centre have a saying: "Nobody ever eats alone." Anyone familiar with anorexia nervosa knows exactly how crowded a small kitchen can be with phantom mothers, fathers, ex-lovers, and doctors holding forth about food, pleasure, health, sexuality, and self-control.

Likewise, any time a parent toilet-trains a child, there are at least two other parents in the room, evoking memories and raising expectations about dirt and hygiene, self-reliance and dependency, compliance and transgression. Karl and Daphne were silent for a while. I asked what they were thinking.

Quite solemnly, Karl said, "I wanted to help her. I should have done more."

I asked if he meant Daphne or their daughter.

"No, I mean my mother. Maybe she loved me too much, but she really protected me. I lived in fear of this man. When he said, 'I brought you into this world, and I can take you out!' you believed it. For years, she protected me, and when I grew up, I protected her. I wish I would have done more for her."

I was surprised by this shift of topic, but Daphne was not. Her face, scornful when we began, softened.

"My mother-in-law is a good woman at heart. She is. I love her, and I can't even think of losing her."

Karl's father had died five years earlier, making his mother the last living grandparent. They spoke of her sweet, daft ways, her perfect pierogies, her love of Rosie. Having her close had made the loss of her own mother a bit easier for Daphne.

Sometimes, however, it made it more difficult. Sometimes it made her miss her own mother even more.

Daphne's mother had been stern but reliable, and she adored Melina's daughter, Lily, her one granddaughter. Daphne couldn't believe her mother would not be around for advice about baby things: rashes, fevers, and pacifiers. She and her mother had just begun to be gentle, even vulnerable, with each other when her mother was diagnosed with breast cancer. Everyone told Daphne to think happy thoughts during her pregnancy, to put sorrow away. Surely it was what her mother would have wanted. But the sadness over the loss of her mom, the memory of this vigorous woman wasting away, was still there, ready to tumble out.

"Two crybabies!" she said. "I thought we were talking about toilet training!"

It was no accident, this little detour. It was very important to be upset about such things. Working out this grief might well help them think more clearly about parenting. We could certainly devote more time to talking about Daphne's mother's death and about how best to take care of Karl's mother. And as for Rosie, was it time to try something new?

It was time, they agreed. Daphne felt they should talk together with Rosie, and that Karl should make it clear that he, too, wanted her to use the potty instead of diapers. They would offer an extra story at bedtime as a reward.

This led to immediate changes. Rosie began to get the idea, and the hours of screaming stopped. Karl had let go of something, a part of his own childhood, perhaps, and his daughter did not hold on to her babyish ways so fiercely on his behalf. Daphne, less panicked at the problem of filling the void, was able to think more constructively about mothering.

•   •   •

Karl dreamed: *I had bought a Walkman.*

I asked for thoughts and associations, and he could tell me only that he had seen one while shopping and wanted to buy it to use at the gym. Again, I had some thoughts that I chose not to voice. (I wondered if he wanted to "*Walk*, man!")

I asked Daphne if she had any thoughts about this first dream of his. *No.* Her smile had a trace of condescension, but she did not criticize him. She asked if she could tell her own dream:

> *I had written something down, and no one could read what it said. I don't even know if I could read it.*

I asked if she had any thoughts or feelings about the dream. She did not. I invited her to take a minute to think. She said she was drawing a blank, which was unusual for her.

"No one could read what it said," I repeated. "Maybe not even *you*. Anything come to mind?"

She stayed quiet and pensive. "No," she said.

My first thought was that the dream expressed a wish to remain mysterious—not to be too quickly understood. Perhaps she was feeling exposed or misread by me, or by others.

Karl said it reminded him of something she had said the other day.

"You said, 'You don't remember things I tell you. I should write everything down for you.' Also, Daphne likes writers. We have a neighbor who is a retired journalist. Maybe the dream is for Walter. Maybe youse two could figure out the writing." Daphne laughed with delight. She said:

"He's right about both things! I did say that to him yesterday. And it's true I admire writers. To me, someone who can put things into words. . . . It seems so powerful. Me, I love learning new words, and it bugs me when Karl says 'ain't' and 'youse.' He could care less. The neighbor is an older guy, but I have to admit that when I talk to him, I think: Wouldn't it be nice to be married to someone who would be so intellectual? He could, like, pull you up with him."

"Not drag you into the gutter like me!"

They were both in a light mood and able to talk freely about something that had long been a sore point. Daphne felt deeply disappointed in herself for not marrying a man better educated than her, someone who could "pull her up" and be more showoffable as well. Karl, she said, was a man who could talk of nothing except wrestling. And of all sports! Football at least involved strategy, and many basketball players were well-spoken. But wrestlers were brutes and everyone knew the games were fixed. Daphne, who had tried so hard to improve her vocabulary and keep up with current events, was stuck with this television-guzzling, pretzel-popping slouch.

This form of wounded self-esteem is the subject of Richard Sennett and Jonathan Cobb's classic, *The Hidden Injuries of Class*. A subject underinvestigated by psychologists, class status influences everyone's self definition. Karl, knowing that his wife considered him a living reproach, tried as hard as he could, at times, to appear philistine. When an evening with friends turned to talk of the news, Karl would sulk and ask if he could turn on the television. One night, friends invited them to see a movie that happened to have subtitles. He complained through the entire picture, so that no one could enjoy it. We talked about finding better ways of standing up for himself. We talked about why Daphne needed a husband to be better educated than herself. Why had she not finished college?

Daphne blamed her parents. From her earliest years, they insisted that boys alone should attend universities because girls just got married and had babies. Furious at the unfairness, she simmered quietly as her brothers got their bachelor's degrees, while she worked in an office. When she saved up enough to attend two years of night school, no one in the family showed interest. In her mind, all this could have been set right by winning an intellectual husband.

I was moved by this conversation, and by Daphne's dream about writing something that no one, not even she, could understand. In contrast to my initial reflection, it seemed to have something to do with wanting to make a mark, even if she did not yet know what it was. She had often described herself as too emotional, as lost in her feelings. Some would say she was dreaming about a new relationship to the world of language and the symbolic. It would not have been surprising had she brought in a dream about babies. Daphne had dreamed of writing.

The dream and the discussion that followed led us back to the question of education. Family size aside, did she want to return to college at some point? No, Daphne said, she had never really enjoyed it. She continued:

"And that is why I can't fill the void with work. I mean, sure, I'd love to fill my life with an important job like yours. If I could be a doctor or a lawyer or something, I would do that in a minute. But if a person can't stand to be in a classroom, and refuses to take a menial job. . . . Well, I've said all this before."

She mentioned that she had been tested at one time to determine if she had a learning disability. That wasn't it. At twenty, she could have pushed herself to study. The moment had passed.

Daphne and Karl entered their next session with big smiles. They had good news: Karl had had a "major dream."

"No more Mickey Mouse stuff," he said.

I was in my parents' house. There is a lavatory on the second floor. I am having sex with a girl from work. She is Gail, who is married to my boss. I am worried someone will come in.

He added that Gail and her husband were leaving the area soon. I asked him to tell me anything else he could about the dream. He said that Gail was a pretty blonde, attractive in a totally different way from Daphne. All his life, he had wanted beautiful women to chase him. Daphne, as striking as a movie star, had been the only one.

He wondered if he would go the rest of his life making love to this one person. The dream was just that, he said: a fantasy of being with someone else. He added:

"I don't think I'm speaking out of turn, here. Daphne and me, we're happy together in bed. At least we were. I'm sure she has thought the same thing, haven't you?"

"I don't mind you saying that," she replied. "I have to admit, I think about it, too, what it would be like. . . . I'm not going to run out and find out. But you do wonder."

I asked what he thought the lavatory was doing in the dream. He said it made the whole thing secretive and exciting, but also frustrating.

Why the boss's wife? He didn't know. Nor did Daphne. A boss and his wife could easily represent the parental couple, making it an Oedipal dream. What had been Karl's experience as a sexual being in his family?

"The setting could be anywhere," I said. "But in the dream you're in your parents' house. What about that, Karl?"

Karl said his parents never told him anything about sex. His father was tall, and Karl was a late bloomer, so the father never missed an occasion to refer to him as "the runt." This, we imagined, was an expression of jealousy over Karl's being the mother's favorite.

Daphne said she saw Karl's father as a "castrating" type of man. He seemed to want to make his son feel like nothing.

"Sometimes," she said, "Karl says I act like his father, tearing him to shreds. He's right, too, and I feel really bad about it."

This was something we had worked on earlier in the therapy, and it is an area in which I find Lacan's formulations helpful. "Castration" is a very important Lacanian term—different from but also related to Daphne's usage. When Lacan referred to the importance of both men and women accepting our "castration," he was referring to the fact that none of us is psychologically or sexually whole. Except in the case of psychotics who actually believe they are God, we are all radically incomplete beings—divided by our own unconscious processes, which often seem to have the upper hand. We are speaking beings, empowered but also doomed through language, since we can never say exactly what we mean. Only those who accept the fact that we are all, in this sense, "castrated" have the capacity to love. Those men and women who assume for themselves some kind of phallic completeness have no chance at intimacy. In Lacanian terms, what bothered Daphne was that Karl's father—and she herself—could act as though Karl were the only castrated being while they, themselves, were complete. They "tore him to shreds" to prove their superiority. It was something Daphne wanted to stop, for his sake and for hers.

Daphne went on to say that her own parents were strict and disparaging about sex. A premarital pregnancy would have heaped shame upon the family, and so her mother had emphasized the dangers of sex, not the pleasures.

Daphne and Karl were sitting close together, knees touching. The air crinkled with pleasant tension. I broke the long silence to ask what they were thinking. Daphne said they had cuddled in bed the previous night and tried some foreplay, and that it was very nice. But there was no intercourse, because he was afraid of getting her pregnant. She, for her part, refused to use any kind of contraception. This was not a religious matter, but a practical one. Together they gave a short history of the miseries they had shared with the pill, IUDs, diaphragms, foam, and condoms. "Please be aware," Daphne addressed me, "that I once offered him a vasectomy, and he refused."

Her sententious tone made it sound as though she had offered to perform the operation herself. Karl may have heard it that way. He was afraid the procedure would destroy his potency.

They were pleased to report during the same session that Rosie was doing well. She had gone to playschool and enjoyed it a lot. She made friends, and she spoke up when she needed the bathroom. Although there were still occasional accidents at home, there were none at school.

The following week, Daphne came in with two dreams. In the first:

Rosie was peeing standing up, like a boy.

And in the second:

I was dressed in a beautiful blue sequined gown, going to a party, or perhaps a convention.

I asked for her thoughts or associations. Peeing standing up? "All I can think of is that we've had potty training on the brain for so long. The second dream, I don't know."

Karl asked if he could add some thoughts.

"To me, if you take the two dreams together, it's like the two parts of her mind. She is still of two minds. She's got kids on the brain, no secret. Maybe she is thinking of having a boy this time. Maybe she thinks a boy would be easier. And second, she would also like to be out in the world doing something special, out there in the public eye."

I turned to look at Daphne. I will remember the look on her face as long as I live. She had pressed the palms of both hands into her cheeks and stared at him. It was a look of tender curiosity, of tickled, sweet surprise. She had married a smart man after all!

Daphne could scarcely speak for laughing and crying.

"I can hardly believe he's doing this! It's so intellectual. And he's good! I mean, what he says rings true. I even said to my sister the other day, 'Karl can do what Deborah does!'"

Karl can do what Deborah does. It was my turn to light up like a lamp.

"It's true, Karl, isn't it?" I said this because I couldn't dance on the table.

"What! Did youse really think I couldn't learn this stuff?" he said. "I like it. It's very interesting."

"I thought you'd think it was goofy," she said.

"No, I think *you're* goofy," he deadpanned. "Dreams are very serious things. Dreams are OK."

"What if he puts you out of business, Deborah? I mean, I'm just kidding."

They held hands and looked at each other, and seemed to be making little private jokes.

I was thrilled that she didn't need me to be the keeper of the magic. Karl was rising to the occasion.

Daphne returned to the dream itself. She never would have decoded it, she said. She kept thinking, "What is my daughter doing peeing like a boy?" She hated to admit it, but she would love to have a son. "You are supposed to want a healthy baby—boy or girl—and thank God for that." But in her heart it wasn't so simple.

"If I had a boy, it would be the first in the family." This was something I hadn't put together. Melina had a daughter, and her brothers also had daughters. Daphne wanted one more chance to win this particular contest. Giving baby clothes to the neighbor had signaled she was leaving the race. And why was it so important to have a boy in the family?

"Because boys have certain advantages," she said. "No matter what people say, it's still a man's world." Karl intervened: "No, we're trying to change that, right? Rosie can be a doctor, or lawyer, or plumber, or rock star, or whatever she wants, right? Maybe a wrestler."

Daphne nodded.

This is a difficult subject for many parents, however, because irrational notions come into play. When stated, they can sound callous or superannuated. I remembered the privileges Daphne's brothers enjoyed. Their names were "James" and "Peter" but she referred to them as "Zeus" and "Apollo."

"They were treated as gods, yes. They didn't have to do anything; they were just adored. I always had to prove myself the loyal daughter. The boys could cut school, smoke cigarettes, have sex, go to college. Melina and I did the housework and had a curfew. When we grew up, we had to help with every medical problem my parents had. They didn't even like to complain when my brothers were around, so as not to upset them. And their wives treat them the same way."

Somewhere, not far from the surface, lurked the desire to produce the privileged character she could not be.

How did Karl feel about having a son?

"I was relieved to know Rosie was a girl. In the sonogram room I said, 'Thank you, Lord!' I just think girls are better, less sneaky."

Daphne suddenly had the thought that Karl's explanation did not go to the heart of the matter. He was probably afraid to have a son because of the relationship he had with his own father. Karl said that if he had a boy he would want to treat him "exactly the opposite" of the way he had been treated. But there would always be a worry, he said, that he'd end up acting like the old man.

They were so engrossed in the discussion, I could hardly get them out the door that night. I heard them in the lobby talking with great energy about this, and found them a week later in that same spot, as though they had spent the entire week in a deep, satisfying exchange of ideas.

•   •   •

Daphne and Karl were doing well. Perhaps some backsliding was inevitable. Just before Christmas, they came in looking troubled. Karl had bought a gold chain for her from a shady character on the street. She was weeping. It was a "hot necklace," she insisted. It belonged to another person, who lost it to a thief.

Karl argued it just wasn't so. The guy was pawning his own stuff because he was short of cash.

Yet Karl looked ashamed. Daphne labeled the act dishonest, hence gambling, and thus something that should be discussed in his GA group.

He protested that he simply wanted her to have something sensational, and felt inadequate for not being able to spend a lot on her. Perhaps, I said, he was angry at her for years of put-downs. For this kind of gift did seem to carry anger or disrespect.

Karl saw it as wrong, but not as gambling, and he did not want to bring GA into it. His late father was a maintenance man who used to brag about all the cleaning supplies he had stolen from work. Karl figured that as an immigrant, his father felt entitled to do that. Karl senior worked so hard, felt he gave so much of himself, that he deserved whatever he could get his hands on. Those free boxes of tissues and soap meant the world to him.

I asked Karl if he had any idea why he himself would do this, give a kind of loyal nod to his father, at this particular time.

Karl said he did not know, except that he always thought of his father around Christmas. He liked to go to the cemetery, but this year, things had been too busy around the house. He hadn't wanted to ask Daphne to go with him.

"I would have gone with you! Is that what this is about? I want to know what you are planning to do with that necklace. Can you take it back to the guy?"

"Are you kidding?"

"See my point, it was stolen!"

Karl suggested donating the necklace to a Thrift-for-AIDS shop. Daphne said that that idea was the best gift he had ever given her. They agreed to visit the graves of all three parents over the holidays.

It was the first good Christmas they had had in a while. Things were going so well that Karl brought up the question of sex, wanting to use contraception, and even raising the issue of a vasectomy. Daphne was livid.

"Yes, I miss making love, too. Believe me!" she said at our first session of the new year. "But I am not using birth control.

Listen to me, you two! I never lived an exciting, daring life, OK? To me, it's a little bit exciting to go to bed and not know what is going to happen. Maybe he has had enough excitement in his life. I haven't. I am still obsessed, and I want to be obsessed, and I will never give in on this issue!"

Karl did not wait for me to prompt him. He was on the verge of crying, but that did not silence him. His thin lips quivered on every word: "We have been coming here for months now, and saying things are better. They are better: But what are we going to do about this? When I was gambling, I didn't give a shit. I felt I had no future. Now, I give a shit. I can't honestly say that I want to raise another child, so I am not about to take a crapshot."

They were reprising the original battle, still causing pain, but also speaking more clearly, more fully. I noted that although it was a very uncomfortable impasse, it was an impasse caused by the interference of changes for the better. Daphne had lived her life in an overcontrolled way. Throwing caution to the wind could be salutary. Karl, however, wanted to go in the opposite direction. Both were moving toward "health," but each in a way that appeared impossible for the other.

Karl said, "I was going to say we're back to square one. Yet it can't be. Because we're talking more. We're more sad now than pissed off."

I reminded them that change didn't move in straight lines, and that they might need to cycle through this issue a few more times.

By the next session, they were absorbed with their plans to travel to Florida in March. Daphne was nervous, not about the flight, nor about the care of Rosie, who would stay with her aunt Melina, but about her own feelings of taking off alone without her.

Karl described a similar feeling. He said that when they went to the mall for two hours, leaving her with a sitter, Rosie would greet them like they had been gone for a month. "I'll be down there knowing she's asking for us, and I'm afraid it will make *me* nuts. Four days is a long time."

We devoted the session to exploring this shared dread. There was a feeling of terrible loss, of something slipping away that could never come back. Daphne smiled, thinking of a dream she had had. It was a bit silly, but she felt she knew its meaning, without consulting Karl or me.

I dreamed my father was making mashed potatoes. Then he was doing what my daughter used to do for laughs—emptying the bowl on his head.

For Daphne the meaning was clear. The dream substituted a baby for a father. If she had another child, especially a boy, it would replace him.

"Bringing a new life into this world makes up for so much that is bad, so much pain. Suddenly, someone depends on you totally. With everyone else getting old and losing their functions, you bring this being into the world who only gets more beautiful every day and more capable. It makes you feel godlike. It's like cheating death."

Karl shook his head, admiring her bumptious eloquence.

Daphne continued. She had always hated it when her mother went away. She began to weep, and I remembered that years back, she had told of a number of separations from her mother. They were not for vacation purposes. Her mother had been ill throughout her childhood, and had undergone several operations, including a hysterectomy at the age of thirty-six. Daphne would wake up in the morning, asking for her mother, and be told by her father to "quiet down." He would say, "She's having an operation, she can't hear you."

He couldn't comfort the children, we decided, because he himself was having a hard time with her absence. He was dependent on her for everything, and was probably terrified of her dying.

Karl, too, had experienced his mother's absence at a young age. There were times when his father "got physical" and started to push or slap her. On several occasions, she chose to leave the house and spend the night with a relative. No one explained these absences to Karl. He could not express his fear or anger at being left behind with "the ogre." Like Daphne, he wondered if he might get left behind for good.

The memories filling the room made it easy for me to make sense of their fears about leaving Rosie home for a long weekend. They were projecting their anxieties onto Rosie, assuming that she would feel what they had felt when left behind. My explanation offered relief. Children often can sense the difference between a situation in which parents are going away on vacation and going away because of illness or victimization.

"It makes sense, what you're saying," said Karl. "We have to be giving off a completely different vibe. Rosie knows we're OK."

They left the session laughing about how they hadn't needed all that travel insurance after all. Daphne had asked her doctor for some Valium, and now felt she wouldn't take it. A teetotaler, she said she might, however, need to have a drink on the plane.

"It's been done before," I said, and wished them a wonderful holiday.

•   •   •

The day after their return, Karl and Daphne entered my office tanned and relaxed, saying they had enjoyed every minute of their holiday alone, and that Rosie was doing fine. She was now, to everyone's surprise, completely toilet-trained. Instead of regressing while they were away, she was keen to show everyone her new big-girl behavior.

Karl asked, "Ain't you gonna tell Deborah the other thing?"

"What other thing?"

"You know, that we're going to bed."

Whereupon they laughed uproariously. Yes, they had resumed their sex life down in Miami Beach. She and Karl had agreed to use condoms, realizing they were taking chances.

"I don't wanna be celibate the rest of my life," he said. "And if we have another kid, so be it. We'll manage, I guess."

Daphne looked at him lovingly and reached out to hold his hand. I asked for her thoughts and she said she had noticed her desire for a second child diminish while they were away. When I asked her to explain, she was quick to say she wasn't ready to give up that part of her life. But she no longer felt the need to rush out and get pregnant. She was grateful for their happiness and did not want to jeopardize it. And despite his faults, there was so much about Karl she enjoyed.

"He is loyal. He is the kind of man who could spend four days on a beach surrounded by twenty-year-olds in bikinis and still make you feel *you* are the one he's looking at. He looked great with his big muscles, walking into the ocean. I would catch him looking at me, and even that would get me going. . . . And I have to say one more thing, you know, because my family was ridiculous about sex, and I felt so uptight as a young woman. I expected sex to be a burden, a wifely duty. But Karl . . . made sex wonderful for me."

I looked at him, fully expecting him to shrug off the compliment, or perhaps to thank her. He uncrossed his arms, studied the floor and said softly:

"She did, too. She made sex wonderful for me, too."

• • •

Karl started the next session by bringing up the chore wars. He did more housework than most guys, and still she didn't appreciate it. She had to supervise, analyze, criticize everything he cleaned or cooked. Daphne didn't deny it. She turned to him and tried to explain that although he did a lot of actual work, he did not do the "planning." It was she who ended up organizing their trip: packing for them and for Rosie, confirming the flights, arranging for someone to care for the dog.

I have heard many other wives and mothers express this very thing. It's the mental energy involved in thinking ahead about the household and everyone in it that is onerous. Daphne gave examples of times she had backed off, only to have important things left undone.

They devoted three sessions to this issue. They were really listening to each other this time, teasing more and blaming less. The resolution they came up with by the end of the third session seemed fair and workable. It was during the end of this session that their smiles of satisfaction led to a long silence. It lasted perhaps ten minutes—a therapy eternity. I hesitated to speak because the silence felt chosen and pleasurable. Some therapists believe that the very goal of this kind of work is to increase the family's or the couple's capacity for reflection, for "reverie." This was a pregnant pause, I thought. And I followed my own train of associations. . . .

Sitting there, I realized what was going to happen: they were going to have another child. They had used therapy to clear a psychological space for a new baby. She had been desperate to have a son, in order not to lose what Karl couldn't give her. He had been desperately afraid of a son—of having a child who would turn him into his father, thus destroying him. They were having sex again and, given the way they felt about condoms, would soon discard or misuse them. They had tried for a couple of years to get pregnant the first time, but then, following surgery to remove a cyst, Daphne became pregnant immediately. Given her family history, she felt confident about being fertile enough at forty.

A baby would be lucky to come into this family in which people could listen and talk, in which extended family members were cared for, in which people made each other laugh and interpreted each other's dreams.

As we were nearly out of time, I broke the silence, asking if either one of them wanted to say anything. Daphne said calmly, without looking up:

"I start working May tenth."

There had been no preamble to this news. Daphne had simply found a part-time job as the receptionist in an office. She seemed pleased. She hastened to say that this did not mean she would never have another child. It simply wasn't on her mind these days.

So much for my clinical intuition! Sometimes a pregnant pause is only a pregnant pause.

I asked if she knew why she wasn't "obsessed" any more.

"I really couldn't say," she replied. "But I feel much better. I hated that feeling. It was like going crazy."

· · ·

It was late April when we said good-bye. Daphne remarked: "I have such a different feeling saying good-bye to you this time. The last time I felt terribly sad—that I would miss you awfully. But this feels natural. I don't know. I suppose if we get in trouble again, we could always come back, right? Unless you move. But even if you move, I guess we could always jet out to wherever you are. . . . "

I was touched by her thoughts, both about being ready to leave me behind and also about feeling empowered to find me if necessary—indeed, to "jet out" for a session.

Karl's eyes welled with tears as he thanked me.

"It sounds sappy to say: 'Thank you for saving my marriage.'"

It sounded lovely.

We shook hands. They promised to drop me a card in the fall.

Four months later, Daphne called about an insurance form. She was eager to tell me she had quit her first job for a second, better one. She was now the receptionist in a large law office. So pleased were the partners with her performance, they were offering to train her as a paralegal. Karl picked up the extension:

"Deborah, this is the most perfect job for her. Get a load of this: She's learning all this legal knowledge and boosting her confidence. She's nicer to Rosie, too."

Was there anything in it for him?

"It's like watching *L.A. Law* to hear her talk about her day. And I like having the extra dough, too."

I couldn't help asking if they were still considering another child. Daphne answered first:

"Definitely not. I can't even remember why I wanted to do it."

I was very curious about how she herself understood the change in her desire. She had, not so long before, insisted on the right to be "obsessed."

"What changed your mind, Daphne? Do you know?"

"It's Karl." she said. "He's my friend, now. I'm not lonely anymore."

They told me that they still told their dreams to each other, something a lot of couples continue to do after therapy. They mentioned that Karl had done well in a weight-lifting competition at his gym.

Working out and watching television were still his only hobbies, which continued to disappoint Daphne. He simply would not get interested in her version of culture.

Therapy had not made quarreling obsolete. They still bickered about the old things, they said, and just as passionately.

Porcupine love such as theirs is at least never dull!

The Loebs, I imagined, would always be both tender and prickly. They loved each other, but not as "kindred souls" do. She liked discussing world news; he felt the family was world enough. She ached for a trip to Europe; he, for more time in the den. They were mismatched, and content to be.

Same bed, different dreams.

2   CHRISTMAS IN JULY

IT WAS JUDITH KAPLAN'S pediatrician who contacted me about her.

"A medical phenomenon" is what he called his eleven-year-old patient, whom he labeled a *superlabile diabetic.*

The word "labile" comes from the Latin *labi*, meaning "prone to slip." The blood-sugar levels of superlabile diabetics rise or fall drastically, inexplicably. Worse still, the patient whose blood test shows the need for thirty units of insulin may inject ten times that amount and produce no change in level.

Most physicians now believe that one key to diabetic control is the management of stress. A kind of medical code word for all things psychological, stress can override the body's natural chemistry to an astonishing degree. The problem is that the causes of stress, particularly in children, are often far less obvious than its dangerous effects.

Judith was a case in point. According to her doctor, she was the oldest child and only girl in a "stable, loving, truly great family of six." In third grade, she was diagnosed with ordinary Type I diabetes, and at first she managed her illness remarkably well. Unlike some children, Judith never complained, not even in the beginning. Dr. Shapiro described having watched then-eight-year-old Judith pull the dietary instruction book out of her mother's hands so she could study it herself. Mrs. Kaplan had administered the insulin injections for the first two years, then Judith took over at age ten. By fifth grade, diabetes had become a completely private affair. Far from taking on the role of the handicapped child, Judith became her mother's right hand at home and every teacher's helper at school.

Six months before her pediatrician phoned me, something had gone terribly wrong, and no one knew why. It started one evening when Mrs. Kaplan asked Judith to finish bathing her three-year-old brother. She refused, saying she felt sick. Judith tested her blood and realized she needed insulin. An hour later, however, her levels had not come down, so she injected more. When even the additional insulin produced no improvement, her parents, close to panic, took Judith to the emergency room.

Judith received an intravenous line for hydration and more insulin, and was stable. When the doctors quizzed her about her regimen, she admitted she had eaten more than usual at a friend's house and had forgotten to test herself. She was sent home with a lecture about junk food.

Six months later during a routine check-up, Dr. Shapiro became alarmed. Judith had not had another crisis, but her numbers now looked dangerously erratic. She also seemed depressed. He asked if she were having problems at home or at school. *No.* He told her that kids her age had new pressures that could throw off diabetic control. Was she arguing with her parents? Did she have a crush on a boy? Was she nervous about menstruation?

Judith shook her head: none of those things applied to her. She did acknowledge "worrying a lot," but declined to elaborate.

She insisted that with more effort she could get her blood levels back to "perfect."

Later that spring, Judith was rushed again to the emergency room. The doctors were so shocked at her blood sugar that they tested the insulin she was using to make sure it was still good. Her baffled parents were sick with concern. That's when Dr. Shapiro told them about our clinic, which specialized in the psychology of stress-sensitive diseases such as asthma, epilepsy, and diabetes. I had been on staff for four years at that point, and had treated a number of diabetic children. For most, the stressors—poverty, child abuse, the absence of family—were immediately obvious. Judith was more enigmatic. Although her parents had balked at what they called "psychiatric involvement," they were, at this point, ready to try anything.

Dr. Shapiro confided to me: "I have known this kid all her life. She tends to be studious and serious, but not like this. It could be the illness that's causing depression, but I don't think so. She's having nightmares, but won't tell me any content. My guess is she would open up more to a woman. I told the family I knew someone who would be perfect for them. They should pull Judith out of school to see you if they need to."

The next call was from Mrs. Kaplan. I offered to meet them that evening or the following day at noon. I asked to see not only Judith and both parents but also her siblings for at least the first session. This was clinic policy, and the reason was simple. Since the 1970s, research on children's psychosomatic disorders has identified the family as a potential source of stress and, also, an excellent locus for therapeutic intervention.

At my request to see the entire family, Mrs. Kaplan cleared her throat a couple of times. She was happy to bring the other children along if I insisted, but felt that her very busy husband should be excused. I had already heard this objection so often

in my professional life—fathers being too busy for therapy—
that I did not belabor the point. I simply said that Mr. Kaplan
would need to attend. Mrs. Kaplan vowed to do her best and
accepted the following day's appointment: Friday noon.

At the stroke of twelve, Pauline, the receptionist, phoned
my office.

"Rabbi Kaplan and family are here to see you, Dr. Luepnitz."

No one had said anything to me about a rabbi.

A consultation that seconds before had struck me as fairly
routine was suddenly fraught. The last time I had treated the
child of a rabbi, I had committed a serious gaffe. After walking
out to the waiting room and shaking hands with the patient and
her mother, I offered my hand to the father, who extended his
index finger and looked away. I remember to this day the con-
founding power of that gesture. I had no idea what it meant, nor
how to ask about its meaning. As we proceeded back to my office, the rabbi had walked behind me and whispered gently, "Just
so you know: Orthodox men don't shake hands with women."

I had not known. The results of that therapy were salutary:
the child got well, and the parents were pleased with the work
we did together. Nonetheless, our early sessions had remained
awkward, and I was keen to do better now with the family in
the waiting room.

I went out and shook hands with Mrs. Kaplan, a small
woman with dark circles under her gray eyes. She was stroking
Judith's hair gently. I shook hands with Judith, thin and pale
with beautiful reddish-gold braids that were coming undone.
She was holding her three-year-old brother, Sam, on her lap.
Judith wore the medical emergency bracelet that diabetic kids
routinely wear, but it looked twice the size of her wrist. Her
glasses, similarly, were about to slip off her tiny nose. The word
that came to my mind was "wizened," an odd word for a child.

I took a few steps in the direction of Rabbi Kaplan, not extending my hand but inclining my body toward him, in a gesture that resembled something between a Buddhist bow and a *petit mal* seizure. A short, energetic man with light-blue eyes, Rabbi Kaplan stood up, offered me his hand, and said a few words to me in Hebrew.

"Excuse me, Rabbi?"

He looked at me and blinked twice.

"I'm glad you could come on short notice," I offered.

"The older boys are not here," he remarked. "They're in school."

I lowered my gaze as we walked back to my office and noticed that Mrs. Kaplan had a significant limp in her right leg. Once we were settled inside, Judith said she needed to use the bathroom, and was excused. Her father, peering at the Easter decorations the patients had made for my desk, chose that moment to say:

"I get the impression that you are not Jewish."

It was *déjà vu* all over again. The last time a rabbi said those words to me in a session I had blurted out something like "I'm sorry, but I'm actually Catholic." That would not be a hard act to follow.

"Rabbi, it seems you were expecting a Jewish therapist."

He nodded. I informed the Kaplans that with our large and diverse staff, it was certainly possible to match them with a different provider, if they so desired. They turned to each other, spoke in Yiddish, and it was again Rabbi Kaplan who addressed me.

"Judith's pediatrician, who knows her well, told us you were Jewish. Since she has never seen a psychologist, we thought it would make her more comfortable, yes. Is it essential? No, of course not."

There was no smiling or joking about this mistake. I suspected the parents themselves would have been more comfortable had I been of their faith.

I said I would be very happy to work with them, but that they should feel free even after our first session to request a transfer.

"No," the parents said in unison.

"We will see you," said Mrs. Kaplan. She got up to pull Sam away from the toy-box. Again I noticed the stiffness in her leg. Judith returned, and her mother spoke to her in Yiddish. She nodded. I was feeling excluded, but didn't want to say so. If Judith felt uncomfortable with me, I doubted that she would let on in front of her parents. I would ask to see her alone in any case.

I raised a question to the family about how Dr. Shapiro had explained the purpose of our meeting.

"Are you asking me?" said Judith.

"Why don't you start," I replied.

"Diabetes has four factors," she said, "food intake, exercise, insulin, and stress. And since my other factors are fine, Dr. Shapiro says I must have stress and need to talk with you to figure it out."

"Well said, Judith," I remarked.

"And the parents are needed to give input, I take it," said Mrs. Kaplan.

"We've found that seeing the whole family is extremely valuable in understanding stress, yes."

I posed several questions about what they had been through during the previous six months.

"It has been difficult and frightening, as you can imagine," said Mrs. Kaplan.

Sometimes families come to therapy with a theory about what has gone wrong—a theory they may or may not have shared with their physician. I asked the question point-blank. It was Rabbi Kaplan who answered that it was a "mystery of mysteries." He had heard of diabetic children who became rebellious in adolescence and stopped taking care of themselves. Judith, he said, was a child who was rarely angry, never defiant. She was a superior student, worked very hard at her music lessons, and showed maturity beyond her years.

Her mother spoke next. The doctors asked if anything catastrophic or unusual had happened in the past six months. Mrs. Kaplan had told them no: No one had died, or been in an accident, thank God. She turned to her daughter.

"Judith, I must ask you again here. And please tell us exactly what you feel. Are you unhappy at school or at home? Has a teacher been unfair? Has anyone, God forbid, hurt you?"

"Has someone offered you drugs?" asked her father.

Judith was not irritated by these questions as some adolescents would be. She simply said, "No."

"There was an incident about girls being rude to her in class one day. But that's it. Maybe you should tell the doctor about that, Judith," said her mother.

"That wasn't so major," said Judith.

I asked if she would mind telling me anyway. She said that their teacher had asked the class to choose a movie they could see together as a reward for finishing their tests. The other kids wanted to see a comedy, and she had suggested something serious. They laughed at her suggestion.

"I remember you were upset by that, Judith. If those girls are a continuing problem for you, we need to talk about this. Maybe something should be done," said Mr. Kaplan.

"No way. That was just a . . . misunderstanding." Judith rolled her eyes, looking for the first time typically adolescent.

I said it was often helpful to pinpoint exactly when a problem got started. When did Judith feel she had moved from normal diabetes management to a situation out of control?

"I can't really say," she replied.

"Roughly speaking," I added.

"I just don't know."

"Well, did the problem start during summer vacation last year, or closer to Christmas?"

I stopped while everyone in the room over the age of three reacted to my inapt choice of holidays.

"Did the problem start closer to summer or *winter?*" I pushed on, feeling foolish.

"Somewhere in between," she said.

Rabbi Kaplan intervened at that point.

"Things got bad in October. That was the first emergency-room visit."

"The numbers were already not good in September," said Mrs. Kaplan.

"I would say the problem started in October." His voice had picked up an edge.

"The emergency-room visit was the fifth of September. I am the one who calls the doctors."

They were interrupted by Judith's knocking over a bowl of marbles on my toy-shelf while reaching for a tissue. Never had forty glass spheres created more havoc. When Judith bent down to pick them up, her father urged her to sit back down and answer my questions. Mrs. Kaplan shot up to grab them away from Sam, who had embarked on a tasting, then roller-skated back to her chair on the ones under her feet. Again, no one cracked a smile during this little drama. They were all overwhelmed by the problem at hand.

I attempted to take some family history, but I didn't get very far as the Kaplans clearly did not find my questions relevant to diabetes management. I found out that they had lived in Israel for a while, that Judith had been born there, and that they had a fairly large extended family living in Philadelphia.

I turned to ask Judith if she had a theory about what had caused this change in her condition. She began to cry, and so did her little brother.

"All her brothers are worried sick," said Mrs. Kaplan. "The fact that they're not here doesn't mean they don't care. They care very deeply."

"I know, Mom," said Judith. "I'm just afraid of having to go into the hospital. I would miss school, and be with kids I'm not used to. I have promised since the *beginning of the year* that I would help Mrs. Schwartz organize the science fair. And who would take the groceries to the Horowitzes? I don't want to be in the hospital. I think I'll be fine from now on."

"You have been saying that, Judith, and it's not your fault, but you are not yet fine."

I asked if I could see Judith alone for a while. The parents looked long at their daughter. As I always do in situations like this, I asked them if Judith had permission to say anything she wanted, without worrying about getting in trouble. (Kids sometimes feel torn about "squealing" on their parents.)

"Yes, of course she does!"

As soon as Judith and I were settled in an adjacent room, she looked more comfortable.

"What my father said to you was a Shabbat greeting, that's all. It's OK that you're not Jewish. Our family doesn't discriminate. I think we all felt a little upset about coming here today because we're not used to seeing psychologists, but that's all."

I thanked her for her comments. Judith was the kind of young person adults love: reflective, articulate, helpful.

My opening gambit was something about diabetes being a difficult challenge in life. But self-pity was not on Judith's agenda.

"Diabetes is no big deal, usually. It's not like having cancer or something."

"Dr. Shapiro told me you learned to manage your blood levels in no time."

"Thank you. My family eats kosher, so I was used to eating carefully. Sometimes we bring our own food on trains and things."

"The injections—"

"—aren't horrible or anything. You just change the spot on your belly each time so you don't get sore, that's all."

Reminding her that I wouldn't repeat anything she told me without her permission, I tried to get Judith to describe what was bothering her. I brought up the night terrors, but she said she didn't know what they were about. She would just wake up cold and frightened.

"Nothing bad has happened *per se*. I just seem to worry a lot."

"What about?"

"I don't really know."

"Your health?"

She looked slightly exasperated at my purveying of the obvious.

"*That* we already know!" she said.

"Can you tell me more?"

"I worry about my family, I guess."

"Explain, please, Judith."

"My parents work very, very, very hard for us. They would do anything for us," she said, starting to cry.

"Yes, you have hard-working and devoted parents, and . . . "

"I don't know."

"Sometimes hard-working parents get irritable and they argue. That can be upsetting to kids. What about . . . "

"My parents argue sometimes. And it upsets me. But I'm not afraid they're going to divorce or anything."

"What do you do when you are upset?"

"I try to be helpful. I play with my brothers."

I asked what it was like to have three brothers. Judith said it was fine, but when I asked if there were anything she would change about her life, she said it would be to have a sister.

"Someone to play and study with me."

I asked again about school and friends. This time she was ready to elaborate.

"I love my school, and my friends are good. But I am very religious, and a lot of the kids are very secular. They're really into being 'cool.'"

The "cool" kids, she said, were crazy for boys, rock stars, and clothes. "Things that don't matter so much to me. Oh, I almost forgot to tell you the most important thing! Miriam, who is a college student and family friend, has moved to Chicago and we miss her, but mostly I do because she used to tutor me in Hebrew, just as a favor to us. She is so great, Miriam, so brilliant, and we all love her. My brother David studies with my father at night, but I don't have anyone to study with."

"Do you ever study with your father?"

"No, because I have to help Mom with the little kids. She has a bad leg. She had polio when she was a little girl, and she gets tired going up and down steps."

"Do your parents know how you feel about wanting someone to replace Miriam?"

"I think so. But right now they can't afford it, and I'm not going to just say, 'Hey! Give me a tutor this minute!' You know, it would be, like, so selfish."

At this point, she fell silent again. I tried to query her about being selfish, but she was starting to shrug off my questions. I asked if she would mind doing a couple of drawings for me before we rejoined her parents.

Drawings offer clues about children's fantasies. They are particularly useful when the problem is urgent and the therapist can't count on months of sessions during which those fantasies might unfold.

Judith seemed relieved at the prospect of doing something besides talking. She drew carefully for the next ten minutes, erased a lot, and handed me the pictures. I suggested we rejoin her parents and Sam.

"Well?" said Mr. Kaplan, as though Judith and I were a jury returning with a verdict.

I said that we had had a good conversation, and that I wanted to continue it the following week. Reluctantly, they made another appointment.

"Please remember, Doctor, with all due respect to you. Our single goal is to get Judith on track again, and not to do in-depth analysis," said her father.

"To tell the truth," added Mrs. Kaplan, "we weren't sure if this consultation involved one appointment or many."

I let them know that it was impossible to do this work in a single hour. I guessed we would need at least five to ten sessions, but that I would accept the goal of getting Judith's diabetic management back on track.

"Can you give us some advice based on what you learned today?" asked Mrs. Kaplan.

The truth was, I couldn't. There was no advice, no set of impressions I could offer at the moment. But her request was certainly reasonable. They needed to hear something from me, obviously.

"Judith's medical condition has stumped her doctors, and we know it's a serious thing. Dr. Shapiro feels this is a problem requiring a team approach. Now I'm on Judith's team as well, along with you and her teachers and the medical staff next door. If Judith needs to go to the hospital again, I will be called. If you should have questions for me before we meet again, please phone me here or at home."

The parents nodded politely and smiled. I showed them out and collapsed into my chair to think. It had been a tense hour for us all. They were a captive audience, present only at the urging of their doctor. On top of that, I was not the person they were expecting to meet.

Everyone who seeks therapy brings a desire for and a resistance to change—a *yes* and a *no*. The Kaplans expressed their resistance by refusing to bring their other children, and by using a language I didn't understand.

Their desire for help was also clear. They had shown up on time, listened, talked, asked questions, made another appointment. My heart went out to them as to all parents with sick kids. The long-term consequences of uncontrolled diabetes can be catastrophic. Four hundred Americans die each day from the disease, and tens of thousands suffer complications such as kidney failure, blindness, and circulation problems leading to limb amputations. The Kaplans had no way of knowing if their daughter's medical crisis had passed, or if this were just the beginning of a downward spiral.

According to some analysts—including the late Serge Leclaire—the therapist must take into account his or her own resistance. My resistance had spoken up for itself loud and clear. Asking a Jewish child about a Christian holiday was my unconscious way of saying: "Give me another family today with a background identical to mine so I can simplify this complicated and life-threatening problem!"

Fortunately, my commitment to help far surpassed my resistance. I admired the Kaplans for following through on the pediatrician's instructions (not all families do), and I viewed our differences as a chance for learning.

I liked Judith. I appreciated her thoughtfulness and her verbal adroitness. She struck me as one of those kids who know that something has gone emotionally haywire but genuinely do not know why.

"I know I worry, but I don't know what about. . . . "

Psychoanalysis takes it as a matter of course that we can know and not know something at the same time. Whether or not Judith was uncomfortable seeing a therapist at all, or seeing me in particular, she had opened up more to me than to her pediatrician. Some therapists would have chosen to do individual therapy, working on her fears, fantasies, and behavior without seeing the family at all. But in general, the younger the patient, the more likely I am to do family therapy. A suicide attempt by a seven-year-old can scarcely be comprehended or treated without family work. Teen-agers, on the other hand, have complex lives of their own, and many request therapy for themselves. Because adolescents are in an in-between time of life, I usually hold some sessions with them alone and others with the family.

Judith was mature in some ways, but not in others. I looked closely at the pictures she had drawn. Although she was verbally precocious, her drawings were immature. She used stick figures where most adolescents would try to sketch flesh and bones. What caught my attention first was the house she had drawn. She had depicted sturdy foundations and a front door with a large door-knocker, but the windows were tiny. A small chimney belched a cloud of dark smoke half the size of the house. If the drawing indicated her family's need to let out steam or clear the air, then the Kaplans would be like many other families that therapists call "psychosomatic." Freud, of course, theorized a century ago that people sometimes use physical symptoms as a replacement for speech. He also noticed the fact that families play a part in the formation and maintenance of individuals' symptoms. In "The Case of an Obsessional Neurosis," he wrote:

> This family plan stirred up in him [the patient] a conflict as to whether he should remain faithful to the lady he loved in spite of her poverty, or whether he should follow in his father's footsteps and marry the lovely, rich, and well-connected girl assigned to him. And he resolved this conflict, which was, in fact, one between his love and the persisting influence of his father's wishes, by falling ill, or, to put it more correctly, by falling ill he avoided the task of resolving it in real life. . . . The proof that this view is correct lies in the fact that the chief result of his illness was an obstinate incapacity for work which allowed him to postpone the completion of his education for years.

The important contribution made by the family therapy movement in the 1970s was one of clinical technique. Freud treated individuals only, but family therapists invited the entire family into the consulting room. The symptom-bearer was called the "*identified* patient," signaling that the true patient was the family. In early research on psychosomatic illness, family therapists found that sick children improved when they were separated from their family, only to return to medical crisis when they were sent home. Researchers determined that the children in those families were containing or absorbing the family's emotional strife, especially the parents' marital conflict. From this perspective, Judith's recent, mysterious diabetic crises were probably a way of resolving a family conflict or of commenting on something going on in the family. The question was *what?* I thought about the moment in the session when the parents disagreed about the month in which Judith's crisis began. The air crackled during that exchange. Judith did not take sides, nor had the disagreement between the parents escalated, possibly because Judith spilled the marbles. Was it her role in the family to create distractions when the parents were at odds? When we were alone and I raised the question of her parents' arguing, Judith had been quick to say that she didn't worry that they would "divorce or anything." I wondered if she did indeed worry about this and, if so, whether or not there was any real cause for concern. These bits of information were enough for me to formulate questions, but not enough to share an interpretation with the family.

I have seen families drop out of treatment after feeling attacked by clinicians too eager to tell them the truth about themselves. The question I ask myself when sitting with a family in pain is not "What can I say?" but "What can I say *that can be heard?*"

That afternoon I spoke with Dr. Shapiro. The Kaplans had consented to my sharing impressions with him, and I was eager to do so. I started with the issue of my religious background.

"You were raised *Catholic?* Now, that's weird because I could swear you said you belonged. . . . I even told the Kaplans you belonged to that ultra-reform synagogue in the suburbs. It's too liberal for their tastes, but they said, 'Oh, yes, good, any Jewish therapist would be fine for Judith.'"

We had a good laugh. He had simply wanted to do everything possible to make the parents comfortable seeking psychological help. It was clear that Dr. Shapiro liked the Kaplans—and Judith especially. Nonetheless, I had the impression that he found her decidedly *other*.

"She's a brilliant kid, you know. I only wish my Hebrew were as good as hers. And she loves anything to do with math and numbers. She's what my kids would call a 'math geek.' When I see her in the waiting room doing homework, I want to say, 'Judith, lighten up! Watch a little TV!'"

I told him that she had complained about the kids at school being "too secular." She had always insisted to him that things at school were perfect.

"How many eleven-year-olds even *know* the word 'secular,' let alone use it casually?" He laughed.

"Not many," I said.

I don't know how many eleven-year-olds use that word, but I had. In fact, I had the same complaint about my peers at that age. I preferred Gregorian chant to rock-'n'-roll, and was probably the only member of our parish below retirement age who opposed the English Mass.

I felt reticent to disclose all this to Dr. Shapiro; we were colleagues, not friends. It would be years before I'd tell him my hunch: that the reason he had chosen me as "perfect" for Judith—bypassing five therapists on our staff who shared her religious background—was because of some better intuition. I actually *was* more like Judith than were the other therapists. She and I shared the knowledge of what it means to be passionately religious in a secular, "cool-girl" world.

•   •   •

The family appeared on time for their next hour, and again the older boys were left home to study. The rabbi said that they had tests coming up, and that it simply did not make sense to bring them along. I was disappointed, as the boys were important to the process. It was also a clear challenge to my professional authority.

"I do hope to see them next time," I said.

"Perhaps you could explain to us why you desire their participation, Doctor," said the rabbi.

I made recourse to the much-used word "stress." In order to gauge the level of stress in the family as a whole—the relevant conflicts or pressure points—I found it helpful to see everyone who lived in the household.

Sometimes even grandparents and nannies come to therapy, I said. In addition, it was clearly the case that Judith's brothers were worried about her, and they themselves might benefit from the chance to air their worries and contribute to her healing.

Rabbi Kaplan nodded. I couldn't tell whether he was simply indicating that my argument made sense or was persuaded to bring the boys next time. He asked if we could discuss the topic of stress.

"We have formed the impression, rightly or wrongly, that we are to keep the stress level down for Judith's sake."

It was an excellent topic. Parents sometimes take the physician's exhortation "Reduce stress!" to mean that they should speak in whispers, spoil the sick child, or stifle all differences of opinion. How did they think about stress, I asked, and what had they done about it?

Judith said the most stressful thing at the moment was having to miss study time when her brothers didn't. It was unfair. I asked her parents to respond.

"Judith, explain please," said her mother.

Judith clammed up again.

This criticism, apparently, was new to them.

"Is fairness an important topic?" I asked. I sensed that it was, because Judith had told me her father studied with the boys while she did housework. I didn't have Judith's permission to bring this up in front of her parents, however.

"If David were ill and needed many doctor's appointments, he would be here, and you would be home studying, Judith."

The parents began speaking to each other in Yiddish.

I couldn't tell what they were saying, but the tone seemed fairly heated. Judith started to squirm in her chair. She told me later that she understood only half, because they talked fast or used big words when, as now, they didn't want the kids to understand.

As the parents spoke, I felt drawn in and, at the same time, excluded. It was impossible not to respond to the emotional charge between them, but I was locked out of the content. Perhaps this is what Judith experienced on a daily basis. I had certainly felt this way before with families, whether they were speaking a language I understood or not. One walks a fine line in these situations. A therapist can be both too aggressive and too deferential in steering the conversation. When the parents paused, I asked if they could summarize their dialogue for me.

"My wife was saying that Judith needs some extra compassion right now. This is fine, but to tell the truth, she has lately had compassion *plus*. One reason I wanted to let the boys stay home is that they have been asked to do her chores all week so that Judith could rest. My wife has brought her breakfast in bed every day, and she has just received promise of a new clarinet, all—I believe—in the name of keeping down stress. You mentioned Christmas, Dr. Luepnitz. I have asked myself all week: 'Is this Christmas in July?'"

At that point, Judith leaned over and whispered to me, "Do I get to talk with you alone today?"

If I could revisit that moment with the Kaplans, I would ask Judith to draw pictures in the other room while I talked alone with her parents. Although the question in the air seemed simple—"How should we lower stress?"—I sensed much more happening between the lines. I already knew that in the Kaplan household, women and girls did the chores while men and boys studied. I had learned that this did not sit particularly well with Judith. Perhaps it didn't sit well with Mrs. Kaplan, either. Was her recent display of "compassion plus" a quiet subversion of the family rules, or at least a way of hinting that she, too, needed something extra? If I had sent Judith out of the room, I might have helped them draw out these questions, and added my two cents.

Compelled instead by Judith's request, or perhaps wary of raising a heavily gendered topic with an Orthodox family, I asked the parents to continue their dialogue with each other while I worked alone with Judith. I offered to answer any questions they had before we stopped for the day.

When we were alone, I expected Judith to be forthcoming, but she was not. She surrendered a few words, then stared at the pictures on the walls, blinking back tears. Could she tell me what she was feeling? Was she bothered by the things her father had said? Judith shrugged. She wasn't saying.

Something I often use with reticent adolescents is the game of Squiggles, invented by Donald Winnicott. The therapist begins the game by making a wavy line on a blank page. The child has to finish it, make something of it, and then give it a title. Then it's the young person's turn to draw the wavy line, and the therapist completes and titles it. It is a projective instrument like the famous inkblot test, but more pleasurable for most patients because it's a two-way game.

I explained the rules and drew a wavy line. Judith turned it quickly into "a balloon sailing over a house." She made some dark, jagged lines, which I turned into "lightning over a field." I drew a squiggle that Judith used to make the profile of an old woman. She said, "It's a grandmother crying." I asked about her grandmother.

Judith had a great deal to say. "Bubby," her maternal grandmother, had died nearly two years earlier. She had a wonderful sense of humor and loved being around the kids. Judith had been especially close to her. Bubby loved Judith's writing, and together they would make up stories. Eventually, Judith took to writing little books for her grandmother, and the series of "Bubby stories" now numbered seven volumes. This beloved family member, so cherished for her vitality, her warmth, her perfect challah bread, had been diagnosed with an inoperable brain tumor and died six months later. Judith cried as she spoke and explained to me the custom of sitting *shivah*. As she finished, she took a deep breath.

"However," she said, "That is not the grandmother I meant."

We had only ten minutes left, and she began to speak about her father's mother, also beloved, although "very stern, a little mean." This grandmother was getting old and needed to live with one of her children. There had been discussion of her living with Judith's family.

"I heard my parents talking about it. My mother thought it might be too hard for her in our house with all the steps. But my father said in my uncle's house there were just as many steps. My mother said fine, she is welcome here, and I think my father wasn't sure if 'Nonny' should come or not. But she was going to come, my mother said, and we were going to move rooms around. And I thought my father was glad, but my mother was worried—glad and worried, too, because my grandmother needs assistance. My mother gets tired with so many kids and her bad leg, even though I help. She was saying I could help with Nonny, but then I got sick."

"What happened then?"

"Everyone in the whole family, all my aunts and uncles were saying if Judith is sick and going to the hospital it's not good to have Nonny there. I mean, I don't know if that's the reason. But I don't think Nonny is coming to live with us."

"How do you feel about that?"

"I don't know. It might be good or bad. Good for my mom, but bad for my dad or possibly bad for Nonny, and I feel it's not directly my fault, but it somewhat is."

I asked if she had ever talked about this with her parents. *No.* She had heard her mother say, "How does your father think we will manage? Who does he think will be helping Nonny in the bathroom nine times a day?" Otherwise, she had heard them talking to each other about it, and it always made her upset when she heard her own name mentioned.

I said it might be adding some stress to the family, and that talking can relieve stress. Would she be willing to bring it up in front of her parents? She said she would think about it.

A few nights later, I got a call from Dr. Shapiro saying that Judith was in the emergency room, and that I was free—although not obliged—to come down. He thought I should know that the parents had asked for me.

When I arrived, she was stabilized, and I asked if we could have a family meeting.

Judith apologized profusely for causing this problem and spoiling everyone's evening. I asked the parents if this was typical of Judith. Did she blame herself for whatever went wrong? They said yes. I had a feeling that this was important—her constant worrying, her blaming herself for things beyond her control. I whispered to her a question about Nonny. Had she thought it over? Would she be willing to bring it up now? Yes, she said, it would be all right.

"Judith says it's OK for me to mention that she worries about her grandmother."

"About my mother?" asked Rabbi Kaplan. "Judith, is this true? Why are you crying?"

Mrs. Kaplan asked, "Is this about Nonny living with us? Oh, Judith!"

The parents outlined the story as Judith had told it to me. The fact was she felt responsible.

Judith said: "Nonny should be able to live with us. You told Daddy it would be too much stress on my diabetes."

The Kaplans were surprised by the depth of Judith's feeling about this, but they could see she spoke in earnest. With my encouragement, they explained the situation to her. They had not, in fact, made a decision about her grandmother, and certainly it was not her fault. Her mother called Judith over and held her, and her father spoke very gently, saying it was good she was speaking her mind. It was remarkable, they said, to see her cry like that; she was such a little stoic at home. Judith was due for a good sobbing, I thought. She said little but wept like her heart was breaking.

I asked to see the parents alone in order to learn more about this particular family issue. There is often more to a story than parents are willing or able to say in front of children.

"My mother is eighty-two, and strong willed, and she wants to live with us. I put the question to my wife."

"If my husband wants his mother to live with us, then it's settled. I simply wondered if our house was the best choice since we have so many steps, and also our children are younger than those of other family members. I was thinking it might not be the best thing for my mother-in-law, that's all. After Judith started needing doctor's appointments all the time, it did make me wonder again about the added strain on both of them."

The rabbi returned, "And I said, the steps are a nonissue, because she would be on the first floor in any case. It's true that my brother's children are grown, and that his house has more room now. I have also an unmarried sister who has offered to take my mother in."

I said to Mrs. Kaplan: "I suppose it would be a lot of work for you with four children to have Nonny there. Is that a factor?"

Her husband intervened. "It would be difficult. I could understand your not wanting to say no—I mean your *wanting* to say no. Especially after Judith started needing so much attention. You never told me so clearly how you felt."

I didn't comment on his slip, but I noticed it. It suggested to me that he was hoping for a "yes" from his wife. Mrs. Kaplan started to cry, and said:

"This is a woman who. . . . " She had to collect herself and start again. "My mother-in-law was in a concentration camp. Who am I to call my life 'difficult'?"

The truth was that Mrs. Kaplan's bad leg had been bothering her a lot, but to refuse on this basis, she said, would be "utterly selfish."

The word "selfish" hung heavy on the silence that followed. Judith had used this word in her session with me. These were the two least selfish people I had met lately, and both seemed plagued by the thought that they weren't sufficiently giving.

There were several ways I could have intervened at this particular moment. I could have turned to Rabbi Kaplan and said, "Would you think your wife 'selfish' if she were against your mother moving in?" I was sure, based on his earlier disclaimer, that he would say "no." I wanted to take the moment to call into question Mrs. Kaplan's use of the word "selfish." And I wanted to use the moment, if possible, not only to raise it as an issue but to strengthen my connection with the family. What could I say that could be heard?

For some patients it would be enough to ask, "What's so bad about being selfish?" Indeed, for many members of our culture, looking out for Number One is the *summum bonum*. I wanted to move Mrs. Kaplan to compassion for herself, without sounding like the voice of pop culture. If I ventured beyond the secular and quoted something from the Scripture I know well, it might needlessly underscore our difference.

I had been taught one beautiful short passage from the Talmud, and this, years ago. It suited the moment perfectly, but I felt presumptuous holding forth like an insider. And what if, nervous as I was, I got it wrong?

"Mrs. Kaplan, isn't there a wonderful passage in Scripture that begins, 'If I am not *for* myself . . . '?"

She nodded, and recited the three lines in Hebrew.

Eem ain a-nee lee mee lee?
Uch-sh'a-nee l'atsmi ma a-nee?
V'eem loh achshav ei-matai?

The rabbi's smile was luminous. He was clearly moved as he translated the passage into English for me:

If I am not for myself, who will be for me?
If I am only for myself, what am I?
If not now, when?

Husband and wife looked at me with warmth and respect. Then they looked at each other, and Mrs. Kaplan said to her husband, "Moshe, I need more of your help with—" and again English disappeared from the airwaves.

This time I did not feel excluded. They were talking to each other about things obviously personal. Mrs. Kaplan had taken the topic I raised and used it to ask her husband for something for herself. More help with the children, more support on the matter of his mother, or perhaps simply more recognition for how much she was already doing. I don't know. But of one thing I felt sure—that Judith's improvement depended on their speaking their minds more fully to each other.

"Dr. Luepnitz, are you telling us that this family dilemma caused Judith's life-threatening crisis?" asked Mr. Kaplan.

Events are multiply caused, I replied. But I did think that Judith's recent troubles had to do with worrying: about the family as a whole, about her grandmother's welfare, about how hard her parents worked, about her mom, especially. She was clearly a very sensitive child who took on the distress of others as her own. This sensitive child had also recently lost someone supportive in whom she confided—Miriam. I had noticed also that the first hospitalization coincided with the anniversary of Mrs. Kaplan's mother's death, a loss I imagined to be particularly devastating. (So devastating, perhaps, that she had had to negate it in response to Dr. Shapiro's questions. "There have been no deaths, no accidents. . . . ") It was not long after her mother's death that Mrs. Kaplan had been asked to take in her mother-in-law. In some situations, a new person in the household could attenuate the pain of mourning. However, the elder Mrs. Kaplan was herself unwell, requiring extensive daily care. And difficult as it is to admit, most of us have had a

thought, however fleeting, like the following: If one grandmother had to die, why that one?

Mrs. Kaplan's reservations about the move, her fear of being depleted, her shame about her selfishness, her anger with
her husband for posing the question in the first place—much
of this had gone unspoken. Judith's symptom had the unin-
tended effect of solving the problem. As long as she was in
trouble, it made sense for her grandmother to live elsewhere,
while no one had to take responsibility for saying, "We've decided against it." No one had to seem selfish.

It was a satisfying session, but for me only a kind of beginning. My preference would have been to pick up these themes
and work through them thoroughly over weeks and months. I
might have held sessions with the parents alone, focusing on
communication and mutual aid so that their grown-up anxieties did not slip into the hearts and minds of their children. I
might have worked alone with Judith on the issues Dr. Shapiro
had raised in the beginning: puberty, sexuality, competition,
and anger. Judith's first crisis had occurred just after she refused to finish bathing her brother. What feelings about her
own changing body had that soapy little boy evoked? Also, Judith had reached the "magic" age of eleven, the year that psychologist Carol Gilligan has noted as pivotal for girls. This is
the age when girls are expected to make a psychological break
from their mothers—one that boys are required to make at a
younger age. Girls are supposed to reorient themselves toward
a heterosexual world, preparatory to marriage and motherhood. Given the difficult lives of their mothers, no wonder
some adolescent girls look at them and protest, verbally or
otherwise.

These topics were on *my* agenda, not the family's. The parents had revealed a great deal in the emergency-room session.

Afterward, the windows seemed to close a bit, and I was asked to focus on Judith, and to bring the therapy to an end.

I did. Judith had a good week following her hospital visit. Not only were her blood-sugar numbers good, but she was acting livelier and brighter. When we met alone, she said she felt much better having spoken about Nonny. Her parents had continued to speak of the problem during the week, and she listened at their door. She had fallen behind in her Hebrew studies, and really wanted a tutor. I told her that if she were to speak up in a family session, I would support her.

Judith asked how many more sessions we would have to have. I was curious about her own desire for further treatment. Some adolescents will make it known directly or indirectly that they object to their parents' attempt to rush the process. In such cases, I argue on behalf of the patient, and the majority of parents cooperate. In this instance, it seemed that both Judith and her parents wanted to do the minimum amount of work and return to business as usual.

Before we finished the hour, Judith asked me to give her some tips for lowering stress. I helped her come up with two. She wrote them slowly on notebook paper and said she would post them in her room. They were:

1. Trust parents to handle their own worries.
2. State clearly what I want and be prepared to compromise if necessary.

In the next family meeting, Judith asked for a new tutor and also for study time with her father. Mr. Kaplan said he would be pleased to spend time with her, but that he would discuss the matter first with Dr. Shapiro and his colleagues. He wondered if the doctors would advise her to take it easy for the

moment and worry less about school. I pointed out that, for
Judith, studying was more reward than stressor, and that exams
had never triggered a diabetic crisis.

I made another suggestion. Her brothers had gone from doing no housework to doing all of it when Judith was ill. Would
it be possible to distribute evenly both chores and study time
with Father from now on?

The parents said it seemed eminently sensible.

Three sessions remained—two with Judith alone and a final
family meeting.

I wanted to be sure that Judith was feeling as strong as she
looked in that last session. She seemed confident and chatty in
those two hours with me alone. She said she had decided she
could worry less about her parents. And why was that? I asked.

"I don't know," she said. "I just get the feeling that they can
take care of things themselves. They never wanted me to worry
about them."

In order to understand this change in psychoanalytic terms,
we again need the construct of projective identification—the
splitting off of painful emotions and "storing" them in another
person. Judith's parents had had a difficult time managing their
grief, anger, and frustration, and Judith had unconsciously "volunteered" to carry the feelings for them. Talking redistributed
the emotional weight. The parents agreed to take on more, and
Judith experienced relief.

She was looking a bit plumper and had better color. I asked
about school, and she said she had done a report on diabetes
for the class. Her classmates were impressed with how much
she knew, and how much she had experienced.

"Remember the movie? When the other kids wanted to see
a comedy and I didn't? The one I wanted to see was called
Shoah, because I had heard my father talking about it with

David and my uncles. They said it was the best movie about the Holocaust, and it takes place in Poland, where my grandparents were. And I felt really upset when they laughed at me, but I don't think they were laughing at me *per se*, but at the suggestion of such a serious movie, and so long a movie, like eight or nine hours instead of one or two."

"I see what you mean, Judith. You know, the first time we talked about this, you didn't mention the name of the movie. Was there a reason?"

"I didn't know if you had seen it."

"Right. Actually, I have seen it. It's a very good and important movie, and indeed very long. Did you mention the incident to your parents?"

"No, because I was afraid they might be really upset about the kids who laughed, and call the school, and then they would just be meaner to me. Because they're all into boys and clothes, and I'm not."

I asked if she had the chance to talk at home about her family's own experience during the *Shoah*.

"My Nonny was in a camp. I know about it. They don't hush it up or anything."

Judith added that this was a topic she used to discuss with Miriam, the friend who moved away. It was at this point that we spoke of ways she could stay in touch with Miriam.

There were several indications that the Holocaust weighed monumentally on Judith's mind. As I looked at her drawing of the house bellowing black smoke, I wondered if she had represented something about her grandparents' wartime trauma. I asked Judith directly if she thought her nightmares had to do with the Holocaust. She said she didn't know.

We can say without a doubt, however, that as challenging as adolescence is for children in our culture, those who grapple

with racism or poverty—or family memories of genocide—
face a much more complicated developmental task.

Judith feared that if her grandmother moved in, she herself
would get even less attention from both parents. The notion
that she had chosen her own needs over those of someone
who had suffered so much had filled her with anxious self-
reproach, just as it had her mother.

"I feel more like I can speak up now, since we started coming here. I was feeling so guilty all the time. But really, no one
thinks I'm bad," said Judith.

On the afternoon of our last session, Mrs. Kaplan phoned
to say that all four children would be attending, but that her
husband would join us late, following a meeting.

At the stroke of six, the receptionist called to say that the
Kaplans had arrived. In the waiting area, I asked Judith to introduce me to her brothers David and Nathan. Sam gave me a
little wave and darted ahead for the toy-box.

When we were settled in my office, Judith announced that
her diabetes was back under control. She began cracking her
knuckles to make her brothers laugh and groan. Judith seemed
less encumbered than before, almost silly.

In order to engage the children as a group, I asked about the
Bubby stories Judith had written. I learned that David had il-
lustrated the books, and that all three boys liked hearing Judith
read them aloud. I liked the titles: *Bubby and the Kangaroo, Bubby
Is a Detective, Astronaut Bubby*. I hadn't seen Judith's lighter side
until now, and I wondered if the stories were as comical as they
sounded. In the session, the children began to talk about their
grandmother, whom they greatly missed.

Nathan, the seven-year-old, changed the subject to ask why
they had come here. As he spoke, I heard Rabbi Kaplan tapping on the door, and I rose to let him in. The kids seemed glad

to see him; he apologized for being late. Wanting to include him, I asked if he would mind responding to Nathan's question about the purpose of our meeting. He said:

"Diabetes is a problem that gets worse when a person is upset, and sometimes the person doesn't even know what's bothering them, so the doctors invite the whole family to come figure it out together, like a puzzle."

It was a fine answer, I thought. I glanced over at Mrs. Kaplan, who was smiling and nodding. We were on the same page.

"So, what was bothering her?" asked David.

Judith laughed. "Everything!"

"Judith is such a caring person, as you boys know, and she was just worrying about everyone, about us and Nonny and Mrs. Schwartz and Miriam, about everybody without end, like the twenty-four-hour store," said Mrs. Kaplan. "She was trying so hard to help us and her teachers that it wore her out."

Rabbi Kaplan looked at me and said warmly:

"Judith likes to be a Good Samaritan."

I was touched by this reference to the New Testament. It felt like a gift. I had shown my acquaintance with their tradition, and he was acknowledging mine. I said to the family:

"It's a good thing, to show compassion, isn't it?"

"It's what we love about Judith," her father said.

"But there has to be a balance between giving and taking," Mrs. Kaplan said. "Between doing and resting."

And the six of them talked about giving and receiving and about why they had decided to divide the chores more equally among them.

"Judith was worrying way too much. Is it possible to worry too little?" I asked.

"Yes," said Mrs. Kaplan, and she pointed to her husband with both hands.

"What's this? I'm needed to worry more? I don't follow—"

"You follow," said Mrs. Kaplan amiably. "You agreed to re-act a little more to things so that Judith and I can react less."

"Oh yes, fine. We talked about that."

"Don't tell me you forgot!" she said, pushing her point.

"I didn't forget, Ruth. I said, 'Yes, we talked about that.'"

"OK. Sorry. You sound very tired."

"Tired, yes, can we move on? Yes?" His pique was rising. I felt the tension move right up my spine.

My eyes were glued to Judith during this exchange. She was fiddling with her hair ribbons and using them as a mustache to entertain Sam. The last time her parents had disagreed in a ses-sion, she had spilled the marbles, creating a distraction. Once again, sparks were flying, but Judith was sitting in her chair like an eleven-year-old girl, not standing over us like a human light-ning rod.

I had a decision to make about her parents' brief tiff—to open it up, or not. I had agreed to the goal of getting Judith back on track medically, and we had accomplished that without probing into their relationship. What was obvious was that they had continued the therapy conversation at home, and that is al-ways a good sign. Even more auspicious was Judith's ability to hear conflict without reacting. I decided to comment on that.

"Judith, you asked me for tips on handling stress. I said the first one was: 'Trust parents to handle their own worries.' It looks to me like you've worked on that one."

She put two hands in the air and said, "Thank you!"

Everyone clapped except the rabbi, who seemed a bit dis-tracted. Only ten minutes remained.

Mrs. Kaplan glanced down at the Bubby books and said she had not seen the latest volume in Judith's oeuvre: *Astronaut Bubby*.

I invited Judith to read from that book, and to show us David's wonderful illustrations.

She did, and everyone clapped, including her father.

Our time was up. They thanked me profusely, and we said our good-byes with the understanding that they could call me again at any time.

No such call ever came.

Henceforward, Judith would carry the diagnosis of ordinary Type I diabetes, no longer "superlabile." Whatever it was that once made her dangerously "prone to slip" had been righted, we agreed, by *talking*.

Psychotherapy doesn't cure all ills. It can't mend fractured bones or fix a damaged pancreas. But it is particularly good at addressing the perilous slips involved in psychosomatic illness, when the body is forced to speak for us.

Lacan's concept of the three registers is helpful here: By this I mean his interlocking circles labeled the symbolic, the imaginary, and the real. According to Lacan, a failure in the *symbolic*—the realm of language and representation—is bound to return in the *real* (in this case, Judith's physical calamity). One could think of our work as addressing this catastrophic slip between registers.

In many families, six sessions' worth of talking would not be enough to produce meaningful results. In a family like the Kaplans, however, in which adults are willing to reflect, take in new data, and change family rules, even a bit of therapy can make a difference. This is particularly true when the presenting complaint is discrete, as with a medical crisis, and of recent onset. Three months of work were enough to reduce one of the famous "four factors of diabetes"—stress.

What, we may well ask, is this stuff? No one has ever seen it, few can define it accurately, but we all know when we have it.

We seem to want less of it and with good medical reasons. Physicians consider stress a compelling factor not only in diabetes but also in heart disease, hypertension, and cancer.

The word "stress" derives from the Latin *strictus,* meaning "compressed." Etymologically, then, stress has to do with too little room and a need to spread out.

This etymology puts me in mind of Winnicott's notion of *potential space*—that intermediate area between the subjective and objective in which creativity and play occur. Psychotherapy is akin to play, according to Winnicott. Therapy takes place neither inside the mind of the patient nor inside that of the therapist, but in some middle area, in the potential space between them.

Judith and her parents were concerned with their household's physical space, and also with the psychological space they needed to provide for various family members. The family used my consulting room—two rooms, actually—to spread out emotionally. A debate formerly waged inside Judith's head moved out to fill the airwaves of the family meetings. This opened new avenues of communication all around. Thus did the Kaplans, and Judith in particular, lose some compression, some stress.

Is it possible to speak of a transference relationship in a therapy of such brief duration? I believe so, although it could not be developed or interpreted. Most of the time, I felt not like a good or bad mother or father with the Kaplans, but like a respected family friend. It's my impression that I played the part of Miriam in the family's unconscious. The parents, although wary of psychological intervention, permitted Judith to confide in me about things personal, as they had allowed her to confide in Miriam. As a teacher of Hebrew, she would have understood the rabbi's initial greeting.

I received a note from the family three months later saying Judith was doing well. Her health was fine, and she had a new Hebrew tutor.

For many years afterward, Ken Shapiro would see me in the hospital cafeteria and say, "Your girl is still doing great!" I was delighted, but continued to wonder about the rest of the family: How would the parents manage their marital conflict over time? Would another child become symptomatic?

Judith, in any case, never returned to the emergency room after the age of eleven.

·   ·   ·

Therapy opens up the imaginative worlds of both patient and therapist. I learned a good deal from working with the Kaplans, and one small example speaks volumes.

Several months after our final session, I reread the story of the Good Samaritan in the Gospel of Luke. The parable, well known, concerns a man who is set upon by thieves and left for dead. He cries out for help, but passersby, including a priest, turn a blind eye. Only one person stops to help, a Samaritan.

> [The Samaritan] bound up his wounds, pouring in oil and wine, and set him on his own beast and brought him to an inn and took care of him. And on the morrow when he departed, he took out two coins and gave them to the innkeeper and said unto him, "Take care of him; and whatsoever thou spendest more, when I come again, I will repay thee."

"Take care of him," says the Samaritan. He delegates the caretaking of the victim to another! The story of the Good Samaritan is not, as I had vaguely recalled, one of selfless, endless

availability, "like the twenty-four-hour store." The biblical passage suggests the ethical possibility, even the ethical necessity of doing a finite amount, engaging others to help, and then moving on.

The story now strikes me as a kind of bookend to the passage from the Talmud, "If I am not for myself. . . . " Both point to a balance between concern for self and a concern for others—a lesson for all times. And for all porcupines.

3 DON JUAN IN TRENTON

You know my motto. "Who is true to one only
is untrue to all others."

—*Don Giovanni*

DAVE JOHNSON rang from the lobby for his first appointment, then seemed to disappear. I stood in the doorway
of my eighth-floor office, checking the clock and shifting from
one foot to the other like a nervous prom date. *Where was he?*
Was he lost somewhere in the building? Had he felt a sudden
change of heart? Run out for a latte?

At a quarter past the hour, flushed but detectably tickled
with himself, Dave turned the corner.

"Holy smokes, Doc, I goofed!" he greeted me.

We shook hands, and I welcomed him inside.

(*Holy smokes? Doc?*)

"So this redhead on the seventh floor," he explained, removing his blazer, "cute as a button, opens the door, her arms
full of folders. I go, 'Is this the therapist's office?' She goes,
'No, that's upstairs. Do you want to use my phone?'"

(Was he making this up?)

"What went through your mind, Dave?"

"Honestly? That I could chat with her and ask her out."

Dave said the mix-up told his life's story. Wherever he went—bookstore, laundromat, coffee bar—he met attractive women eager to engage him.

"I'm not the handsomest guy on the block," he confided. "I can't dance. But I have always had this effect on girls. Even as a little kid, they treated me like the Big Mac."

I looked at him. Dave Johnson, five-feet-elevenish, was wearing an expensive-looking blue shirt with gold cuff links, a Rolex watch, well-pressed khakis, and loafers without socks. He flashed a smile that revealed teeth the color of standard bathroom fixtures, but he was not, in fact, strikingly handsome.

"The effect I have on women is due to my adoration of them. Dave likes to please the ladies, whether it means bringing roses or fixing their personal computer."

When we talked on the phone, I had had trouble under-standing what Dave wanted, what was wrong. That's not un-usual; many people find that first call daunting. I tried again to find out what might bring him from Trenton to Philadelphia—a good forty-five-minute drive—to see me.

"It's not rocket science, Doc. Dave needs to work on your basic issues of sharing, relating, being communicable, and what have you."

He sounded like a man reading his own inpatient chart. Was he crazy or just odd? I asked him to tell me more about himself.

"I'm a veterinarian, like I said on the phone. Usually, I'm a happy, well-adjusted guy. Healthy as a horse. Six months ago, I started to feel like hell. I'm exhausted all the time, achy, with no appetite. I get these headaches, and I started to wonder if there could be something really wrong, so I got checked out by my internist who was able to rule out the heavy-duty stuff."

"What exactly needed ruling out?"

"Your cancers, autoimmune diseases, that stuff."

"Right."

"He suggested I talk to a shrink, and you came highly recommended. The drive doesn't bother me."

"So your two concerns are your physical malaise and your relationships?"

"Yeah. Exactly."

Dave Johnson, age thirty-three, wanted me to know that he had dated many wonderful women in the past few years. His liaisons averaged two to six months, sometimes overlapping each other. The women he dated ranged in age from eighteen to forty-four. He looked down on men who were drawn to a single "type": redheads, slender blondes, or what have you.

"To me, all women have a *quality*," he said, jingling his car keys.

There was something uncanny about this man, in the Freudian sense of being at once quite strange but also ultra-familiar. For a second, I thought he might be someone I had known in grade school.

Dave added that although he'd had his share of one-night stands, he disliked them. He understood that there were women who, like men, enjoy sex for its own sake, but they weren't his cup of tea. He fell for women who wanted commitment.

The problem was that although he enjoyed the intimacy with those women intensely for a short time, he soon felt bored or crowded. Several girlfriends apparently had raised the question of marriage, and Dave felt bad about refusing. But it would be a greater wrong to marry before he could promise fidelity, he said. Although he loved children, he wasn't ready to be a father.

While Dave was easily overstimulated by intimacy, he simply could not tolerate being on his own for long. Like the porcupines in Schopenhauer's parable, he found the pressures of closeness painful; but when he disentangled himself from a woman in order to "take space," he felt completely alone in the world, unable to enjoy his freedom, and desperate for the nearest warm embrace. His account of the problem led to a brief excursus on gender.

"Women deserve better than they get. I respect females more than males. Males are competitive jerks, if you ask me."

Accordingly, as much as he hesitated to try therapy, he would see only a female therapist.

Dave reprised his list of physical complaints and added another, the most vexing: He had lost interest in sex.

"I can get the plumbing to work, but I've lost my drive. That may not sound like a big deal, but it's never happened before. It's kind of spooky."

His physical problems started six months prior to our meeting and three months into a relationship with his current girlfriend, Sylvie. He could see the old song and dance about to repeat. She wanted promises he couldn't make, and he was about to leave her. Dave said he had never felt so bad about ending a relationship. Sylvie's parents were dead, and she counted Dave as her sole protector.

"This girl is so beautiful and so nice. She has this amazing . . . *quality* about her. It will feel awful to unload her."

Wistful as Dave was, unloading seemed to be in the cards. He explained that he not only couldn't see a future with Sylvie, he no longer desired her sexually. They would plan a nice evening together, but after dinner, he'd find himself achy, tired, craving sleep.

I had a hunch about what was going on with the two of them; it was not, as Dave might say, "rocket science." He liked Sylvie not too little but too much. The symptoms were articulating what he couldn't say in words—that the intimacy was painful and depleting. I hoped to slow him down long enough to reflect on the relationship rather than derail it for good.

Dave let me know that his girlfriend saw things the same way I did. In fact, she had urged him to enter couple's therapy to work on their problems, but after some consideration, Dave declined. He wanted out.

In order to avoid thinking about his romantic woes, Dave claimed to be pouring himself into work. His job involved giving shots to cats and dogs, and the occasional surgery. He liked his co-workers and his boss, whom he compared to his father. Dave's father, Joe, died when Dave was eighteen.

"My father was top-shelf. I will never be as good a person as he was."

Joe Johnson was an anesthesiologist who pioneered a new technique, making a name for himself—and a fortune, as well.

"My father was a humble man. He could have run with a fast crowd, but he preferred to be home, not necessarily with us, but in his study. My mother called him 'our father who art upstairs.'"

Dave described his mother as a good person but also a "total flake," the kind of woman who thought the car had broken down when it was simply out of gas. Dave was not condemning her for it. "When you think of how women were raised in those days. . . . "

Neither parent had been unfaithful in marriage.

"My father was a quiet guy. Still waters run deep, you know. Shallow brooks are noisy."

"What would your father say about the situation you're in now?"

"'Give the Don Juan thing a rest, Dave. Time heals all wounds. An ounce of prevention is worth a pound of cure.'"

"Meaning what, Dave?"

"Meaning I have to face facts. Tell my girlfriend where I stand and get myself together. What would be *your* advice?"

I smiled. "What do you imagine?"

"I imagine you'd say, 'I'm not here to give advice, pal, but to help you figure out what the hell *you* want.'"

"How would that advice sit with you?"

"I don't know. But it seems to me that in thirty minutes flat, you've already got the ball rolling. Not bad! Sharma, my internist—Indian fella—told me to interview a couple of therapists before deciding on one, but I don't feel the need to look further. You really have. . . . You most definitely have a *quality*."

I wasn't sure if I should take this as faint praise or lavish condemnation. I decided to chalk his obtuseness up to first-session jitters. Nobody could speak in clichés all the time.

"Trenton is my only other problem," Dave said, standing up and stretching. "I could definitely stand to lose Trenton."

I didn't know what he meant by that, but we were out of time.

Dave made another appointment and handed me his check.

"I think this could be the best thing that ever happened to me, Doc."

I closed the door behind him and found the soft click of the lock reassuring. There was something oppressive about this guy. I wasn't experiencing fear or hatred in the countertransference, as I have with patients who killed their children or fed them drugs, but I was put off. I had a faint urge to wash my hands, to wipe off his gummy adulation.

Paying attention to these thoughts, inchoate and groundless as they must be after a first session, is crucial for therapists. Acknowledging to oneself an initial dislike for (or a strong affection for, or sexual attraction to) a patient greatly reduces the chances of enacting those feelings. Realizing that

I had experienced Dave as fake and ingratiating helped me use the information diagnostically.

Diagnostically, Dave's presentation pointed toward the category of the "false self" or "as if" personality. The person who forges a hyper-compliant façade does so for good psychological reasons related to experiences in childhood. If parents are depressed or abusive, for example, children learn that it is not safe to ask for attention, because survival depends on tracking the adults' moods like the weather. The child gives up on having a spontaneous, desiring self in order to act as the parent to his or her parents. Winnicott said that in these situations, the child's "true self" goes into cold storage and a false, "caretaker self" takes over. Winnicott also believed that smarminess or sentimentality represented "denied hate." Was Dave Johnson, the great lover, actually a great hater? Maybe he did well to leave his women early on; maybe he was protecting them from more destructive impulses.

Maybe I was jumping to conclusions.

His reference to "Don Juan" made me smile. Don Juan has long fascinated students of psychoanalysis who still study Otto Rank's 1930 classic, *The Don Juan Legend*. The character named "Don Juan" made his debut in the early 1600s in *El Burlador de Sevilla*, a play written by a Spanish monk. It is a cautionary tale about the demise of a dissolute nobleman who boasts one thousand and three conquests. In the play's final act, Don Juan is pulled into hell by the avenging father of one of his female victims. This is the story Mozart retells in his magnificent opera *Don Giovanni*. Molière, Byron, and Shaw devoted major works to Don Juan. Philosophers from Hegel to Kierkegaard to Camus have analyzed him variously as the man at war with God, the artist in search of ideal beauty, or the social critic in revolt against bourgeois marriage.

Otto Rank saw Don Juan as the quintessential Oedipal victor. For Rank, real-life Don Juans were men who succeeded as boys in wresting the attention of their mothers away from their fathers. Such victories are usually Pyrrhic, and thus the Oedipal victor grows up hobbled in his adult efforts to love and be loved. Rank made a cogent case for the Oedipal interpretation of Don Juan:

> Clearly the endless series of [seduced women] along with the injured third party characteristic of the Don Juan type appears to confirm this analytic interpretation: That the many women whom he must always replace anew represent the one irreplaceable mother; and that the rivals and adversaries whom he deceives, defrauds, struggles against . . . represent the one unconquerable, mortal enemy, the father.

Ironically, then, Don Juan, for all his love of freedom and contempt for the domestic, has never managed to leave home.

I had seen a number of men in my practice who fit Rank's description. It was too early to tell if Dave, too, would fit, but the possibility was playing in wisps of thought as we met for the second time.

Dave entered that session saying he had felt slightly better during the week, less fatigued and achy. He had told his girlfriend he had seen a therapist who recommended he break off the relationship and try a period of sexual abstinence. She cried and insisted she would wait for him until he was ready. It hurt him to see her upset. He stayed and held her through the night. He hoped she would give up on him.

"Sylvie deserves better. This girl looks like Winona Ryder and has the heart of an angel."

Suddenly my mind went to a more sinister variation on the Don Juan type, a character who figured in a terrible Argentine movie I had seen just weeks earlier. The super-handsome protagonist finishes making love to a woman, then lights a cigarette and taps a button that ejects her through the floorboards into oblivion. She is replaced by a new woman, and the same thing happens. I had watched the movie with an Argentine friend and conversation turned to the question of who needed that button more: women or men.

Sitting across from Dave, I wondered if his girlfriend felt she had been sent bounding through the floorboards, or if she had seen it coming. Knowing nothing about this woman, I couldn't help thinking that she could do better. Dave, himself, seemed to think so. In any case, what was going on in this man's mind that would make him dump a woman in my name? Did he fancy me as some indulgent mother writing to his teacher: "Please excuse Dave from this sexual relationship. He doesn't feel like it today"? I had to comment.

"Dave, I didn't recommend abstinence. I don't recall recommending anything when we met last week."

"Oh, I know, Doc. I was using some poetic license. I didn't want her to think I was cheating on her, and I really do need to be on my own."

The farewell to Sylvie seemed to fling open the door of memory and leave it permanently ajar. In the weeks that followed, Dave recounted his past adventures to me, assuming that I would mildly disapprove, and succeeding, actually, in evoking disapproval. There was the sixteen-year-old bridesmaid at his uncle's wedding, the flight attendant on the trip to West Palm, the only good-looking female professor in the vet school, and assorted secretaries in his office building who relied on his computer prowess and flea-busting skills. He found their lost documents and cured their beloved pets, and so they adored him. A number of these women had abusive partners, whom Dave took immense pleasure in displacing. Rescuing a woman imperiled by another man was his specialty. Mission accomplished, Dave was ready to move on.

I felt a bit like Leporello in *Don Giovanni*, the sidekick who keeps a list of his master's conquests. Leporello was able to deliver warnings to women on that list. I had no such power.

Dave walked in one evening carrying a jacket over one shoulder, his lips pouty as a *GQ* model's.

"Special-looking black lady in the elevator today."

As he described her figure and clothing, I realized he was referring to another patient of mine, and once again I felt protective, although the woman could certainly fend for herself.

The mention of race happened to bring him back to his family.

"I am not a racist. And that's because my parents weren't. In some parts of New Jersey, it's lily white, you know, and people are afraid of Blacks. My father hired Afro-Americans in his office, and my mother welcomed all my friends, regardless of race. Even one of the Ratpack was black."

Dave seemed not to know that "Ratpack" was the name of a group of young musicians whose most famous member was Frank Sinatra. He went on to tell an endearing story about his band of closest high-school friends. These boys played sports and studied together, and were accepted into the homes of the others almost as family members. On Mother's Day, said Dave, each of the four boys went out to buy a dozen roses. First, he gave his own mother three, then he stopped at the homes of his friends' mothers, chatting and offering the gift of three. At the end of the day, each mother had twelve roses. I found this clever and sweet.

"There you go. You probably think, 'That's when all his girl-chasing started.'"

"No. I was actually thinking it was a lovely thing to do."

Dave looked confused. He seemed to need my disapproval. I was interested in knowing whether or not his father sent his mother roses. The elder Dr. Johnson was forgetful in that department. In fact, said Dave, on the evening of his wife's forti-eth birthday, he had fallen asleep in his lab and missed the party.

"You mentioned last week that your father—"

"I hope we're not going to get stuck analyzing my parents. They were—are—very cool people. The problem is *me*."

"The point wouldn't be to analyze them, but to—"

"I know, but I just want to finish telling you about these guys, because they were the best friends I ever had."

Unfortunately, they had moved to different parts of the country. He had no male friends now. He had decided, pretty much, that men were self-centered jerks who only wanted to scam women.

Really?

Feminists are said by their detractors to hate men. Actually, I have never heard men as a group disparaged more vigorously than by men like Dave Johnson.

"All men are that bad?" I asked.

"Gay men are OK. They tend to be more gentle, less mascu-line. Now, of course, you're going to think I'm gay. Is that what you think?"

In fact, a corollary to the psychoanalytic truism that Don Juan is Oedipally fixated is the notion that he is an unacknowl-edged homosexual. Unable to admit his attraction to men, he poses as someone even crazier about women than his straight peers. No doubt, this describes a certain number of "womaniz-ers." However, the fact that Dave had gay friends and was not obviously homophobic didn't convince me his true desire was for men. It was too early to conclude or rule out anything.

In the proceeding months, Dave's sessions followed a certain routine. He would sit quietly for a few minutes, fiddling with his watch, and tell me more about his history with women and, when relevant, about his male rivals. We were working a bit better, I thought. He was telling these stories not to impress or to shock but to make himself known, for he had never spoken so frankly to anyone. I would ask questions and make comments, but the final fifteen minutes of each session felt deadly. He would say at this point that he had "run out of words." Occasionally, he would calculate his loss.

"Ten blank minutes; that's twenty dollars down the drain."

I tried my best to stay attentive during these gaps, but it wasn't easy. The other Don Juans I'd known were riveting. A bit of their randy charm always wafted into the consulting room, keeping things lively. Why were Dave and I so disengaged? One thing I knew: prodding him to talk more or suggesting topics that suited me wouldn't help. Unfortunately, the empty silences were long and getting longer.

I came to realize that Dave was genuinely frustrated about the gaps at the end of sessions. He said he wanted very much to cooperate. He hoped he was "doing it right." He knew that in therapy one spoke of fantasies and dreams, but his fantasies lately were all about vacation, and unfortunately, he did not dream. I reassured him that he did dream, everyone did. He simply wasn't remembering his dreams, and probably would in time. It was at this point that Dave outdid himself by asking:

"Doc, what should I be dreaming about at this point? What do you imagine I'm dreaming at this stage of my treatment?"

This was a complex communication, but I felt exasperated at what struck me as sheer entitlement. I flashed on a biblical

passage I hadn't read in years, in which old King Nebuchadnezzar summons Daniel, the renowned interpreter of dreams,
and demands some dream analysis. Daniel rolls up his sleeves,
as it were, but learns there is one catch.

"The thing is gone from me," says the king.

He requires Daniel first to tell him what he dreamt and,
then, to interpret it.

I told Dave there was no way to tell what a person "should
be dreaming," and that when he did remember a dream, he
might want to write it down. A moment later I realized that
Dave might be telling me something important about himself:
that his own imagination was so impoverished he couldn't quite
remember what it felt like to dream, to reflect, to fantasize. Because free association is another way of gaining access to unconscious material, I again encouraged him to tell me as often
as he could what he was thinking during the long silences.

"Can you tell me what you were thinking just now, for example?"

"Not a thing. Just about work."

"About work?"

"I was thinking about a woman who brought her fox terrier
in because it had worms, and we couldn't figure out what kind.
She finally told me they had had the dog on vacation while hik-
ing in the hinterlands of Guatemala. I couldn't believe that for
three weeks she hadn't thought to tell me that. . . . I told you I
wasn't thinking about anything relevant."

"Is there anything you might be forgetting to tell me, that
might help us understand *you?*" I asked.

"I don't know," he said, twisting his watchband. "I suppose I
should mention the problem of the HSV."

His answer came back after only a brief pause, as though he
had been waiting for me to ask the question in just that way. I

asked Dave if he wanted to tell me his history with HSV (herpes simplex virus).

He had contracted it at the age of twenty-five from an eighteen-year-old woman who did not know she had it. He was devastated by the diagnosis, and briefly considered suicide. He came to see that, just as the doctors had predicted, the first outbreak was the worst, and the first year produced the most outbreaks, after which he would be troubled by the disease perhaps four times a year. Medication had eased the symptoms, and, he said, he was living proof that herpes didn't kill your sex life. I asked how he handled the matter of disclosure to partners.

"One in four Americans has it," was his reply. "In general, I try to be honest."

"In general?" I asked, trying not to sound censorious.

"Some women, you feel that they don't really want to know," was Dave's answer.

Apparently, he thought I was one. Did he mind my asking if he had ever transmitted the disease?

"Twice," he said definitively. "Maybe three times. But we're talking eight years here, so when you think about it. . . . "

When I thought about it, I understood why one in four Americans has the disease.

The outbreaks were accompanied by listlessness and a flu-like feeling. The unwellness he had felt for the previous six months was related to an unusual number of outbreaks—one every two or three weeks. Even daily or "suppressive" doses of acyclovir were making little or no difference.

"I didn't mean to be dishonest with you. In fact, I've meant to tell you. We just never got on the subject."

This is absurd, but not preposterous. On the one hand, to speak to a therapist for months about flu-like symptoms leading to depressed libido and not mention the physical malady involved is absurd. On the other hand, it is the case for almost all of us at some time that the dread of losing face—or simply facing the truth in a new context—makes it difficult to know what we know.

Dave was eager to learn the effect of the disclosure on me. I was glad he had been able to tell me. Perhaps he wished I had guessed it sooner?

"Possibly. But more likely I would have walked. It's embarrassing."

And the abstinence, I wondered, how was that going? He said he was liking it a lot. He had to admit, he had often thought about not having sex—about taking a break. He imagined that a "sabbatical" would bring peace of mind, and better concentration. It was being alone that he found uncomfortable, disorienting.

"If there is no woman in my life, then what do I do at the end of the day? How do I get through work if there is no reward—no lady to wine and dine, and ask about my day? When I'm not with somebody, I'm a hermit."

Thus, one conversation with a woman at the mall would arouse his desire. Almost instantly, he was involved again for a two- to six-month stint.

He had filled the last quarter of the hour, heretofore left blank, with some interesting self-observations: about what was, in fact, his own version of the porcupine dilemma.

Dave was taking therapy seriously, yet I was still distracted by my dislike of him. Did he put me in mind of men I had known in the swinging seventies? Was I simply disgusted at the thought of his infecting women with his sexually transmitted disease? Or was it envy? Don Juans see endless romantic possibilities ahead that the rest of us may not see.

Two months later, Dave reached my door a few minutes early, in time to see another patient, a seven-year-old boy, leaving with his parents. He sat down on the couch and said, "I didn't know you were interested in younger men."

He had made me smile. Dave continued, "You know what Mae West said, right? She said she preferred younger men because they have shorter stories."

I burst out laughing. I covered my lips and collected myself only to crack up again. He had to be the last person with whom I'd associate the giggles.

"That really is a good one, isn't it? I can't even remember where I heard it. It might have been when I was dating Donna, this pretty lady down the shore. She was forty-four when I was twenty-seven."

I didn't comment, but I noted that I was approximately the age of Donna. Perhaps from the start his feelings for me had an erotic tinge that inhibited him in session. As for eros in the countertransference, it was still noticeable for its absence. Certainly, Dave was more likable when he was vulnerable or funny. But the robotic Dave, the "as if" man, was still so present I couldn't imagine any woman finding him attractive. Lord Byron says of his Don Juan:

> . . . *with women he was what*
> *They pleased to make or take him for; and their*
> *Imagination's quite enough for that.*

I glanced at the clock. He had been staring out the window for ten minutes.

"Where are you, Dave?"

"I wasn't thinking anything profound, Doc. Just work again. The day started off bad, but ended up good."

It turned out that the day had begun with an irate client complaining to him about a surgery done on her cat six months earlier by Dr. Sal Curtis. The cat was still limping and miserable. I asked why the owner hadn't spoken directly to Dr. Curtis.

"The pecking order!" said Dave, as though I were some new brand of idiot. This was actually the first I had heard about trouble with the boss. Dave had always described this man as a "great guy," albeit one without "people skills." There appeared to be a collusion among the staff to protect the boss from problems and, if necessary, to take responsibility themselves for any such matters. "It just doesn't pay to drag him into client complaints. He likes to sneak up to his office and nap between surgeries. Whatever. We love him."

"Our father who art upstairs," I thought.

Something different had happened that day. For some reason, Dave had decided not to be in the middle. He had directed the angry client to Dr. Curtis, and afterward stood up for himself and the staff.

"He didn't love the idea—don't get me wrong. The thing was a malpractice situation with a capital 'M.' But he understood what I was saying. People were high-fiving me all day. It felt great."

What felt great had something to do with being true to his principles, and with trusting this man he claimed to love enough to speak his mind. Dave seemed also to have glimpsed something about the function of idealization.

"Everyone says Dr. Curtis has no people skills because he's brilliant. What if that's a big cop-out to leave him off the hook?"

"Right. Sometimes we idealize our superiors because we can't admit to our contempt for them."

"It's not a pretty thought, but it rings true."

Dave started his next session by saying he'd had a great week. He was feeling well inside and out. He said the previous session had worked the cure although, strangely enough, he couldn't remember what we had talked about.

"Not one thing?" I asked.

"No. Except I joked about Mae West. And there was that cute little guy with the Yankees cap, leaving your office. What a sweetheart."

Dave fell silent for a long time. This particular silence felt full. He was not tapping his foot or checking his watch; he was deep in reverie about I knew not what. It was an unusually cold winter's day, and he had kept a royal-blue cashmere scarf around his neck. His dark eyes looked less startled, more relaxed. Free of its usual rigidity, Dave's face seemed quite handsome. When he tugged on the scarf, I got the feeling once again that I knew him from somewhere. He didn't resemble anyone I could call to mind: not a patient, friend, or neighbor. Could it be he looked like some minor actor or television personality? (Dan Aykroyd from the old *Saturday Night Live* came to mind.)

"Where are you, Dave?"

"Nowhere, Doc. I was fading out, thinking of that little boy, or maybe what I was like at that age."

"What were you like?"

"I have no idea. I wonder if my parents would have . . . would my father have come to therapy with me? I can't see him doing this kind of thing. He lived in his head. My mother would have done it, of course. At that age, she was still reading to me all the time. I would do anything to get another story out of her at bedtime. Sometimes I would go in their room and usually they would let me stay. It makes me wonder now how they ever managed to. . . . Anyhow, then he broke his leg when I was ten, and slept in the guest room for a while, and I would sneak into her room. I'd go to his side of their king-size bed and she wouldn't even know I was there until morning. Hey, why are you making me talk about all this Freudian stuff? I told you, I feel great. I'm a poster child for therapy."

"I thought the Freudian stuff was pretty interesting. What about you?"

"It's OK. There's always more to the story, isn't there? I mean, aren't there guys like Woody Allen who stay in therapy for decades? And I don't have his dough! It feels like a good time to cut back, maybe meet once a month—for coffee. I don't know how you work things with your patients; couldn't it be more like friends?"

I chose not to interpret the switch from a memory of replacing Father in Mother's bed to a request to go out with me for coffee. I was pleased to have a chance to begin what some therapists call a "here-and-now discussion" about boundaries with this patient who felt entitled, even impelled, to possess women. Apparently, it did not occur to Dave to wonder if I would want to be his friend. I told him that I never blur the distinction between professional and personal relationships. I did not want to meet as friends, but I did very much want to be his therapist. I was relieved to hear my words come out gently, without an edge.

Something about seeing the little boy in my office had moved Dave deeply. "A sweetheart," he called him, and he remembered himself at that age. What had happened to that little boy, I wondered—the Dave who was animated and contact-craving? Through what process had he moved from spontaneous to stupefied—a man on an emotional hamster wheel?

Something deadening happens to boys in our world, says psychologist Carol Gilligan. Social forces crush boys' inclination to show feelings and to play with girls as friends. Rejecting the culture of competition and misogyny at a certain point means "refusing to be a man," in the words of feminist John Stoltenberg. Don Juanism—the collecting of women—obviously feeds on social forces, not just on familial, Oedipal dynamics. Dave's reaction to the presence of the child left me thinking about these issues for days, and I was eager to learn what he would bring to our next hour.

Dave entered the following session announcing he had remembered a dream—the first since he had started therapy. He had placed a tape recorder next to his bed and had spoken into it when he awakened during the night.

Dave had dreamed of his father. They were washing the car together. In the dream Dave thought, "He doesn't realize he's dead." He awakened feeling extremely sad.

This was the first of several sessions in which he was able to speak about his father—his life, his death, the funeral. Dr. Johnson senior had failed to show up for his speech at a medical convention. Hotel security finally entered the room and found him dead of a heart attack. It was the summer before Dave was to start college. He failed most of his courses the first year, then decided to take some time off. After only two years he had managed to squander his inheritance on first-class plane tickets and a couple of luxury cars. Fortunately, most of the money had been left to his mother. While he felt reassured knowing that he would inherit a certain sum after her death, having to borrow from her from time to time was something he found extremely awkward. Sometimes he would go without, and fall behind in his rent or ask friends for a loan rather than "hit her up again." As a result, Dave said, he often didn't know if he himself were rich or poor. He had survived his father, and would inherit his wealth, but the spoils were remote—impossible to enjoy.

Such is the lot of the Oedipal victor, Rank might have said. He replaces his father and becomes his mother's partner, but at unrecoverable costs. As with many grown-up sons in his situation, Dave's feelings about his father, his mother, and the part he played in the family triangle were so little understood that he couldn't enjoy anything—not even the pleasures rightfully his.

Dave and I did not meet the following week because I was out of town, and I remember worrying about him. Sometimes a short gap in treatment at a crucial moment proves so jarring to a patient that he counters with a hiatus of his own making. There was no cancellation message from Dave when I returned, and he showed up for his weekly session on time. He was quiet and fidgety, though, and returned to the topic of termination.

"I honestly think I'm done. There's not a story left to tell. You've heard about all my girlfriends, all the skeletons in all my closets. I have no more hidden meanings. What you see is what you get."

I decided to take him at his word, and looked at him carefully. Dave always wore a shirt and blazer when he came from work and something casual when he did not. Today was a casual day; he was wearing a light-blue sweatshirt I had seen before. In the low light of my office, I could just make out a pattern above the left-hand pocket. I hoped my eyes deceived me, but no. Against the blue background were, indeed, two minuscule yellow feet.

"What I see is what I get, Dave. And I was just noticing your sweatshirt. Would those be two footprints?"

"Yes," he said. "They represent the size of a baby's foot when it's aborted. It's a pro-life sweatshirt. I'm pro-life."

Dave proceeded to assure me that he was against killing doctors and firebombing clinics; he was no wacko. He went on to state what sounded like a sincere "pro-life" position, weakened only by his habitual use of clichés, which, as always, made it seem that someone had done his thinking for him. He said he was uncomfortable with the conversation because he supposed I was on the other side. It was "all the books," he said, so many books about women that made him assume I was pro-choice.

And if it were true that I was pro-choice? He said he could still respect me, so long as I didn't try to change his mind.

I told him that I wouldn't try to change his mind. I also let him know that therapy often does involve examining one's political and religious beliefs—those that match the therapist's and those that don't.

"Fair enough," he said.

I asked how he came to hold the position he did. Dave told me he had actually once been pro-choice. But then things happened, he said, glancing at the clock and noting we were nearly out of time. "Some things happened, but that is a really long story. . . . "

When I assured him that we would have time for that long story, he asked for a second appointment that week. The only opening I had was the following morning. Dave accepted. He would have to cancel his morning appointments.

.   .   .

How is it that a man can say in earnest on Wednesday at five o'clock that he has told his entire story and, before six, remember that he once had a child who died?

There was, it seems, one relationship that Dave hadn't mentioned. At the age of nineteen, he found himself dating sixteen-year-old Jodie, whom he met at the movie theater where they worked. Jodie was seeing a man in his twenties when she became enamored of Dave, and she slept with him a couple of times. When she realized she was pregnant, Jodie was terrified to let anyone know. She wanted an abortion, but knew her Jehovah's Witness mother would forbid it. Dave also felt abortion was the better option, and was relieved that Jodie did not want to become a mother.

Summer break was approaching, and she arranged to stay with a sympathetic aunt in New York. Jodie ceased contact with Dave during this period, possibly to reconnect with her previous beau. She phoned Dave only in the fall, and when they met, he was overwhelmed to see her six months pregnant. He had been thinking the pregnancy was terminated, and the relationship over. But Jodie's aunt, fearing family reprisal, had refused to help her niece. And Jodie's mother informed her daughter that she would both bear and keep the child. Dave was not to show his face in their home.

Jodie told Dave she was losing her mind, and needed him close to her for strength. They spent the last three months of her pregnancy together, and Dave felt painfully torn. He felt responsible for what had happened, and felt he should support the child. Perhaps, indeed, they ought to marry and try to make it work. Dave's mother felt the girl had set him up by lying about her age and then carrying through with the pregnancy behind his back. How could he even be sure it was his child? Dave was shocked by his mother's lack of compassion. Although he maintained that his parents were not racist, he wondered if Jodie's being half-black had anything to do with his mother's reaction.

Jodie's labor set a record in the hospital. She was physically depleted after thirty-six hours, but healthy. The baby, however, had been in distress during labor, and the doctors did not expect him to leave the hospital. Baby Mike rallied, however, and went home with Jodie after two weeks in intensive care. Defying Jodie's mother, the two young people continued to see each other, Dave sneaking into the house almost daily.

Jodie was depressed and ambivalent toward the baby— sometimes clinging to him for hours, at other times refusing to hold him. Dave described himself as dazed and incompetent during those months. He listed for me the multiple ironies. He was forbidden to act like a father to the baby by Jodie's mother—the only parent who insisted that he *was* the father. He had never wanted anything to do with this child, yet he found himself praying that Mike would survive. The infant had light-brown skin, but Dave occasionally clung to his mother's position that the father was actually Jodie's dark-skinned boyfriend.

"It was . . . fucked *up*," Dave said in a throaty cry.

At four months of age, the baby died, and one month later, Jodie was hospitalized for a suicide attempt. Subsequently, she joined her mother's church and parted ways with Dave. They saw each other only twice after the baby's funeral.

"It was so unbelievably awful," he said, stabbing at the tears in his eyes.

I asked if he could tell me what he was feeling.

"Oh, don't fucking ask," he said. "Not because you shouldn't ask, but because I don't know. It's unreal. It feels like it happened to a different guy, in some parallel universe."

"In order to go on living, you had to erase this hugely important chapter from your life."

"I wonder if you're thinking, 'This guy is the biggest asshole.' I wonder if you'll think less of me. But I'm like relieved, too. I've been sitting on this thing almost half my life! It has followed me around like a goddamned lost dog."

Less of him? I was thinking that at last there was a man, not an android, in the room.

"I feel like I'm finally meeting you, Dave!" I felt sorry for him and for everyone involved, including both grandmas. Dave himself must have felt monstrously alone at nineteen. I wondered if there had been anyone in whom he had confided.

"There was a priest. After the baby died, I felt so empty and guilty. The priest said that Mikey was in heaven with God, so there was no reason for grief. He said I felt guilty because I had wanted her to abort—wanted her to kill my own child. He said God intervened to prevent the abortion, and that I could make up for it by praying, and going to Mass and all. He called me up a couple of years ago, and asked me to join his group. They meet on Saturday mornings in Philadelphia to try to keep women from going into the clinic to have abortions. We don't get physical or anything. We do sidewalk counseling. You know, like: 'Please don't kill your baby. You have other alternatives.' You know?"

I certainly did know. I had stood in front of that very clinic on Saturday mornings for years, sometimes escorting patients through the thicket of demonstrators, sometimes holding the sign that said "This Clinic Is Open!"

Now I knew why Dave looked familiar. He was not a kid from my grammar school, he was the guy in the royal-blue scarf who stood next to the man with the Elmer Fudd hat and the outsized rosary. The latter had a habit of fingering his beads and roaring, "Hail Mary, full of *grace!* The Lord is with *thee!*" And then, to my regular chagrin, "Blessed art thou among *woman!*"

Given that a rosary consists of fifty-three Hail-Mary's, this use of the singular for the plural would work my last nerve before the morning was half over. On one occasion, I actually hurled back: "The *word* is *'women'!* Blessed art thou among *women!*" The clinic director had immediately walked over to chastise me with her usual "No heckling, please."

Had Dave recognized me as the lady who roared back at the man with the big rosary? Is that what he wasn't saying during his many uncomfortable silences? I was distressed. Why hadn't I recognized him immediately? And if I had, what exactly would I have said? It would be two years before we'd return to these questions, but we did so, to good effect. What was important during that emotional session was that he had broken his silence. No wonder he wasn't ready to marry and have a family. I felt new warmth and protectiveness for this young man, who just days before could irritate me impressively. I imagined the suffering of both young people as they tried to navigate the enormous mental shifts confronting them. Will there be a child? Possibly, yes. Then: No, we've decided to terminate the pregnancy. Then again: Yes, we no longer have a choice. Later: No, the baby will die in the hospital. Yes, he has rallied, and will live. A final *no*, after four months.

Dave's history of multiple, indistinguishable flings suddenly seemed more complicated and poignant to me than before. The many endings of affairs he had initiated since Jodie might have constituted a desperate means of psychic survival, of asserting himself over and over against that loss. He would do anything rather than know that kind of pain again.

I agreed with the priest in one small part. I think that having wished not to have the child did make Dave *feel* culpable for the infant's death; this is in the nature of guilt. But my view of what had gone wrong was different from the priest's. Other clergy members might have recommended that Dave do volunteer work for a safe-sex education program or work for reproductive choice, for that matter, so that girls like Jodie would not lose their legal right to choose.

For what seemed like the first time, Dave joined me in pursuit of the past. He wanted to remember the early part of the relationship with Jodie, before the whole dizzying dream unfolded. He wondered who he might have become by now if things had turned out otherwise. He wanted to talk about what he did while she was in New York, about the ways he tried to contact her, about the run-ins with her mother. He had felt enormous dread at the prospect of parenting, and yet he cherished the memory of holding the infant close. He described the night Jodie rushed Mike to the hospital, unable to breathe, and the call that followed, leaving him with a devastating mix of relief and agony at the news of his death. Dave reminded me that his father had died just one year before this happened. To lose a father and a son in so brief a span of time was a lot for a nineteen-year-old to shoulder.

Dorothy Parker once mocked someone by saying that her emotions "ran the gamut from A to B." Dave had been a constricted kind of man, but he changed dramatically at this point. His eyes flickered with chagrin, misery, relief, and rage; an unused alphabet of feeling now marked him.

"Every time we talk about this, it's like my heart stabs itself. I feel sick, even a little nauseous all day. For a while, I was getting better in therapy. My outbreaks had stopped, but now I'm feeling worse. No offense to you, but I have never felt this shitty in my life. I have crying bouts and I've been leaving work earlier every day. I'll be out of a job if I don't pull it together—and fast. This is not going right, Deborah."

I was sorry for him. It was clear that he wasn't exaggerating; he probably did feel worse than he had in his life. But that was the good news. I did not hesitate to give him a little talk about the value of depression.

Donald Winnicott spoke wisely about depression as an achievement. Anyone who has become depressed has reached the limit of the defense mechanism called *projective identification*.

Dave did not forget about Jodie entirely, but he split off his pain and allowed her to contain it. When he mentioned that she had attempted suicide and ended up in a psychiatric hospital, I wondered, in fact, if she had had a nervous breakdown for two.

In the years that had followed, Dave continued to locate his own misery in his lovers, whom he chose for being capable of deep emotion. Instead of grappling with his own devils, he found women who would. He then had the more palatable job of comforting a person in distress.

Projective identification is not always a bad thing. On the contrary, at times we all need to banish overwhelming emotion, or to blame external sources, just to survive psychically. If it becomes our way of being in the world, however, both feelings and judgments are compromised. Failing to get depressed, Dave had grown stolid. As though to keep his feelings in check, he had come to think of the world in absurdly facile terms. Thus, his father had been nothing more than a misunderstood genius, his mother a good-hearted flake. Men were selfish creeps; women, angels with broken computers.

Dave said it made sense to him when I spoke about the value of depression, the importance of it. But the insight did nothing to diminish depression's disabling grip. He was useless at work, and requested some vacation days to regroup. Dr. Curtis asked if there was anything wrong, and when Dave told him about therapy and grieving, the boss was annoyed. He had once granted Dave time off to chase after the Swedish secretary upstairs, but he showed nothing but disdain for this talk of emotions.

"Buck up, boy," said Curtis. "You've got the world by the tail. We've got a lot of work to do in this office. No time for a pity party."

Without the option of taking time off, Dave started thinking about medication. I offered to give him the name of a psychiatrist-colleague with whom he could consult, and we discussed the pros and cons of trying medication. Dave had read about the new antidepressants—the SSRIs—because a number of veterinarians were prescribing them for animals. He knew that decreased libido is a common side effect in human patients, and he wasn't sure he could tolerate that. Dave decided to give himself a month to feel better. If he didn't, he would sign up for "Vitamin P," as his friends referred to Prozac.

Two weeks later, Dave came in with the following dream:

It's pouring rain. A soft, sensuous rain, almost sexual. I have no umbrella. There is lightning, too, but no sound. An older man asks how long I have been standing there. I say, "for four."

I could see from his expression that the dream had not struck him as particularly meaningful. I tried to be gentle, and not clobber him with the question the dream provoked in me.

"Any associations or ideas, Dave?"

"Not a one. What do you think it means?"

"You said the rain felt almost sexual. Could the dream be about sex?"

"Meaning what? That I'm a guy who has sex with no umbrella, no protection? But I've been careful since Jodie."

"Would it be OK for me to ask if your last girlfriend was one of the partners who caught the herpes virus from you?"

"She didn't. Sylvie had it when we met. She told me right away."

"Since you both had the virus, did you feel it was OK not to use condoms?"

"During a safe time of the month, sure. It was a nice luxury, if you get what I mean."

Dave knew that Sylvie was using no other form of contraception, and that she longed for children. This was an egregious risk, given everything that had happened after the last unplanned pregnancy. There he was, taking that chance with her, while denying he was doing any such thing. I asked what would have happened had Sylvie become pregnant.

"I don't think I ever thought about it," he said, shrinking into the floral armchair, and finally sitting on both hands. "I mean, technically, it could have happened. I mean, I know how babies are made, so of course it crossed my mind. . . . It would have been pure hell. I don't know that I could have survived another unwanted-baby scenario. Sylvie wanted a kid bad, but she always said she wouldn't be a single mother. I'm pro-life, of course. I guess I would have left it up to Sylvie; it's her body. I just never . . . you know? Am I making any sense?"

"Not yet," I said, too crisply. This was a bit of countertransference cheekiness, provoked by my experience with antiabortion people who become *de facto* pro-choice when their own well-being is in question.

When we are unable to mourn the past, we cannot leave it behind. Too often, we decide—consciously or not—to repeat the past, either because it's all we know or else to get it right the next time around. Freud called this *Wiederholenzwang:* literally, the compulsion to repeat. But Dave did not end up repeating the first trauma, and we know why: a symptom developed. Illness came to the rescue. For no clear medical reason, he began having herpes outbreaks at six times his usual rate, and the medicine that had always provided relief in the past (and that would again in the future) was suddenly providing none at all. The HSV outbreaks, with their accompanying loss of interest in sex, kept him from potential disaster: becoming a father again before he was ready. In order to banish all longing for Sylvie, in order to silence his own questions about the predicament, he had simply sent her away.

Dave cried for Sylvie, for the best relationship he had ever had. The thought that she had found someone else was devastating, but he had to hope she was happy.

I asked Dave if we could continue working on the dream. (I felt I had landed on it like a ton of bricks.) When he expressed eagerness to do so, I asked if he could say more about the "soft, sensuous rain."

"I have always liked to take walks in the rain. It's a romantic thing I've done with all my girlfriends."

I asked about "no umbrella."

"I don't like umbrellas, OK? I guess in high school you weren't a real guy unless you walked around without a coat or anything, regardless of the weather. But even now, I don't carry one. They never seem to work; they break in your hands. Just like condoms."

"What about 'lightning with no sound'?"

"I don't know. As a kid, I liked lightning until the thunder hit. Then I was terrified."

"What about 'an older man'?"

"I couldn't see his face. I don't think it was someone I knew. He was just a man wearing a Burberry raincoat." To which Dave added, "My father wore Burberry raincoats year-round."

"What comes to mind about the question 'How long have you been standing there?'"

"Nothing. Not one thing." (Later that week he remembered his father punishing him by making him stand up at the dinner table and apologizing for making a mess.)

"The answer in the dream is 'for four,'" I said.

"Again, nothing. For four. Forty-four? That would be the age of Donna Miller, who I dated at twenty-seven. She looked a lot younger than forty-four, and yet the age difference still freaked me a little bit. She literally could have been my mom."

"For four," I repeated, in case he had more to say.

"Nothing. Actually, when you said it just then, it sounded like stuttering. Fff-four. I don't remember this, but my mother told me I stuttered for a brief time in kindergarten. She asked my father if I should see a speech teacher, but he said no, I'd outgrow it. And I did."

I asked about the feeling tone in the dream.

"It was nice and soothing at first. The older man made me kind of nervous, like he was checking me out. Yet I was glad he was there."

Dave's associations converged around basic Oedipal themes. A father figure is "checking him out" as he engages in some romantic activity (walking in the rain). The answer he gives to the older man alludes to an older woman—someone who "could have been" his mom. The actual stuttering that had apparently occurred around age five may have reflected anxieties about being so close to his mother. The reassuring presence of the older man in the dream perhaps bespoke relief that he wasn't his mother's only love. Dave's associations reminded him how pleased he was to have both a mother who would worry about his stuttering and a father who had faith in his resiliency.

Dave was exhilarated to hear so much emerge from his own associations. Above all, these vivid memories of childhood filled him with longing.

How he wished his father were alive! Something made Dave feel that if his father had lived, none of this would have happened. He knew very well that his father had been more than a distant genius, but who could tell him who his father was? Who could say what that man had wanted from life, from marriage, from his son?

I watched him cry, and imagined wrapping him in my attention. If there weren't answers to his questions, the questioning itself would prove salutary.

Dave's third and final year in therapy was the most challenging. Grieving for his father, for Sylvie, for the baby, and for his own lost innocence produced a desire to know more. Dave spoke first with his mother. He drove to Vermont to spend time with her, doing chores and asking about his father. She described the man she married as creative but driven, a quiet man who had not become withdrawn until his own father died, when Dave was five. Dave was, in fact, named for this grandfather, whom she described as a "*bon vivant*." She recommended that Dave speak to his aunt—his father's twin sister and confidante—who lived on the other coast.

Aunt Bert Johnson—a clinical social worker, unmarried, cat-owning, and large-hearted—welcomed him. Although she acknowledged being close to her brother, she insisted that no one knew him. It was her impression, however, that he had suffered depression throughout his adult life. He hinted at things, he brooded, he left clues. Help was not a concept he understood.

Dave's grandfather, in contrast, was gregarious and playful—to a fault, she said. "He was a ladies' man, Dave, and everyone knew it. There were rumors of his having a slew of illegitimate kids. I believe there was really only one—a boy. We were not allowed to ask questions, even as adults."

Dave noted the irony that such an outrageous man as his grandfather could have had a son like Joe, such a straight arrow, so serious, the most serious man in America.

His aunt stayed quiet and then said, "Well . . . maybe not quite so straight-laced as you think."

In going through Joe's papers after his death, Dave's mother and aunt had happened on four or five large cartons of pornographic magazines. His mother had shrugged it off, saying, "I didn't know about all this hot stuff. I suppose that's how men are." Bert had been more curious, and found that they were stacked alphabetically and in perfect chronological order. Most of it was "run-of-the-mill" stuff, she said, but there were also dozens of gay men's magazines.

"Maybe it wasn't his!" was Dave's first response. His aunt smiled again.

"He had a little stash in his briefcase in the hotel the day he died."

"Dad was gay? Just what are you telling me?"

Owning a bunch of magazines didn't prove much about anyone, she said, but it had put a question in her mind. Was he attracted to men? Maybe that was why he never felt good about himself, despite his accomplishments, and why he had cut himself off from his colleagues—mostly male—at the hospital. As for Dave being a lot like his grandfather, Bert remarked that certain behavior seems to skip a generation in families. Or perhaps Joe had turned Dave into his own father out of longing. Joe was proud of his son, she wanted him to know. He felt Dave was good-hearted, hard-working, and a charmer. She said he liked Dave's reputation as a heart-breaker. He didn't mind it, he might have even fostered it.

It is commonly assumed that a man who philanders had a rogue of a father. There are families where this is true. However, of the twenty or so Don Juans I have treated, only two had such a history. This counterintuitive fact highlights the inadequacy of theories that rely on "modeling" to make sense of family psychology. "Monkey see, monkey do" explanations are of limited value in interpreting the lives we live. Only a grasp of the unconscious and of processes such as projective identification can explain, in the words of Aunt Bert, how behaviors can "skip a generation."

Dave returned from California looking like he had aged a couple of years.

"Was my father a homosexual? Could I be gay? Some people think it's biologically determined, you know."

"Let's talk about this," I agreed.

"I honestly don't think I'm attracted to men. I might notice a guy is good-looking or something."

Dave felt we should make this subject a high priority. He also decided to go and speak to one of the physicians—an openly gay man—who had worked with his father years ago. The colleague in question was very kind.

"I knew about your dad, Dave," he said. "Joe was a huge support to me in the department when I came out. He didn't confide in me about his own issues until a year or two before he died, but I always knew. It broke my heart because I could see he loved your mom. He had such a capacity to lose himself in work. There are gay men who live their whole lives like that, never coming to terms with themselves because they don't want to hurt their wives and kids."

It was not the idea of a gay father that overwhelmed Dave as much as the idea of a father with a secret life. Joe was not the absent-minded professor whom people liked to tease, but a man torn by his own desires, intricately calibrated, sensuous. Why, Dave wanted to know, had his mother not understood that he was suffering, whether from depression, sexual confusion, or something else? How could she have lived with a man for twenty years and not recognized his troubles? It was as though he had lost his father a second time.

How differently my patient began to speak in therapy! Dave, who often opened his sessions with a gambit like "What's up, Doc?" walked into my office one evening with a single, very interesting word:

"Anesthesiology!"

"Yes?"

"Anesthesiology, Deborah! My father devoted his life to helping people get numb."

Joe was the last target of his resentment. His father, like Sal Curtis, had worked hard not to feel things. Even when in the room, he must have seemed absent to his mother. Dave decided he would try again to speak with her, and found her more open than before.

"I did everything to get Joe to talk about his dark moods," she said. "It was lonely for me, too, you know. I realized there were . . . personal things . . . that bothered him. But don't forget the world was a different place then. We got married in 1954. Do you think people were busy talking about this kind of sex, that kind of sex? You kept things inside. And I still say that, compared to most marriages, we got along."

Dave felt a new respect for her. She was someone who had lived with what were now obvious disappointments with a quiet dignity. And after her husband's death, she had moved house and developed new friends and interests, all on her own.

In therapy, Dave was trying to rewrite his family story based on the new information. He was in kindergarten, he said, when he began to sense that his mother preferred his company to his father's. And no wonder. Joe Johnson, by all accounts, was emotionally distant, while Dave was attentive and fun. Joe withdrew still more when his own father died. Dave was five when his father lost his father. For Joe, unable to deal with the loss, it may have been just as well that his wife seemed besotted with their son.

A five-year-old boy who can win a woman away from a thirty-year-old man will be undaunted by future rivals. From the standpoint of the unconscious, he has already landed the finest catch of his life. Such boys often long for a parent who could say, "You may not possess your mother; she prefers me, and I, her." There is safety in such defeat. It spares the child the fear of reprisal, and also the dread that invariably comes as he wonders if he could satisfy her adult needs and desires, unfathomable as these must be to him.

It is for this reason that the "Don Juan" figure in myth, literature, and life appears to us as someone who is trying to get caught or punished. He shows us through word or deed that he longs for someone to check his hubris, to say, in effect, "There is a force greater than you."

Together, Dave and I considered the idea that, failing to find a forbidding father, he was driven to become a father himself. In the new triangle of Dave, Jodie, and Mike, the son died and the father lived. Perhaps therein lay some kind of unconscious settling of scores. The priest had functioned as a sententious presence for a short time, but he and Dave never became close.

Dave wasn't ready to stop his research. Suddenly, he wanted to reconnect with everyone. He tried tracking down Jodie, and learned she was living in Alaska. She sent only a card saying she was doing well, and did not want to revisit the past.

He also found Sylvie, who was, predictably, still angry and mystified by his behavior. She had finished her degree in engineering, and had also had a few years of therapy. Despite an abiding affection for Dave, she was feeling "just a little too healthy" to get involved with him. He asked if they could be friends.

Above all, Dave became a man who could abide his own company. He began going out at night to listen to music and, although lonely, was not compelled to pick up women. The first couple of evenings, in fact, he described himself as "dazed." He would sit in a dank New Jersey jazz club close to the stage and stare at the musicians, barely touching his beer. As weeks passed, he became aware of his surroundings. There were interesting women and men around—lovely women alone, women with friends, women in couples. He couldn't approach anyone. What followed was a period of burning and persistent fantasy. In our sessions, he would describe a simple conversation he had with a waitress, recounting in detail the attraction, describing her deep, plummy voice, and the way he wanted to touch or kiss her. These descriptions were utterly different from the jejune tales of his early therapy. Dave was discovering sex.

During this period in the treatment, Dave's interactions with me took on a warmer, lightly eroticized cast. It's true that earlier on he had let me know he liked older women and had, in fact, asked me out for coffee. This new phase was different. He expressed curiosity in me in ways that did not suggest he wanted to gain control of our relationship or end it. One evening he commented on a new outfit I was wearing, and he imagined I was meeting my partner for a late dinner. He imagined further that I had been married a time or two to highly successful, intellectual men, and that I had lately chosen someone different—a handsome carpenter, perhaps, or an artist. His comments were thoughtful and not fulsome. He was able to make these remarks without a demand or expectation that I reveal details of my personal life. I felt at last that there were two adults in the room and that the person addressing me was a man. And a charming man, at that.

Dave decided to go with a friend to a gay club. He talked to men there—he even danced—but he had to agree with his gay friend that he was "overwhelmingly straight." All of this became grist for fantasy, involving strangers, former lovers, and the images in magazines. While he found what he called "dirty pictures" exciting, they always lost their erotic power after a brief period of time. He felt as though his gaze drained them dry, after which they would elicit first disgust, then anger, and then guilt. This sequence of reactions he compared to the memory of sleeping with very beautiful women.

"I would feel totally infatuated with a woman and want desperately to sleep with her, and then enjoy it a lot if I could get her in bed. But the next morning—it sounds awful to say, but the last thing in the world I wanted to see was that woman's face! The very same features that I had thought were so irresistible the night before—her eyes or teeth or whatever—would turn me off. Then I would feel shitty for having those thoughts, and feel sort of paralyzed. I'd hang in there for a while, hoping they would lose interest before I had to make it obvious that I was needing to be alone."

"I remember your saying you disliked one-night stands. You would stay for months at a time with someone."

"I hated it! I just couldn't be the shit that other guys were, so I had to be nice, but believe me, nine times out of ten, I wanted *out*."

Dave apologized for sounding crude and sexist, and I told him he sounded more real than he had in his creaky, tin-man persona of three years back. This highly experienced lover was beginning to reckon with his own brutality, indifference, and doubt. It slowed him down, to be sure. When finally he asked a woman out, he felt he was starting from scratch. What if she could read his thoughts, and find him confused and needy? What if he couldn't perform? He told me that therapy had made it impossible to lie any longer about his sexually transmitted disease, so he now had to face more sexual rejection than ever before.

Remarkably, he didn't blame his father, his mother, or even me, the messenger. He accepted this new vulnerability as proof of his existence. This is how it would be for a while as the changes settled in. . . .

"Incidentally, how exactly did therapy make it impossible to lie about your STD?"

"I don't know. It just wouldn't work."

"Do you have any idea how that changed?"

"Maybe I'd hear your voice saying, 'What the fuck do you think you're doing?'"

"That would be *my* voice?"

"You never said that. I don't know. I just couldn't do it. When I was diagnosed, I wanted to die. How could I do that to somebody else just to get laid easier?"

Five months later, he met an attractive veterinarian and established a friendship that became sexual. They had been dating for six months when we decided to set a date for our last session. Dave wasn't demanding displays of devotion from this woman. They weren't talking about marriage; they were having fun.

Three years after starting therapy, Dave Johnson left Trenton. It was a town he had never liked. He remained there because he couldn't imagine leaving Sal Curtis, the father surrogate. He moved to a larger metropolis, taking a job with greater responsibilities. He was determined to create a workplace where everyone could speak up, and where the bosses, too, were accountable to clients.

His sex drive returned as strong as it had ever been, and his herpes outbreaks were no more or less frequent than they had been before the crisis.

To Dave, these were huge signs of progress. To me as well, but the most redoubtable was his change in language. By the time we said good-bye, I could swear he hadn't used a string of Dave clichés in over a year. Was this all in my head? Maybe I was simply less bothered by his style of talking because I liked him more.

A friend of his had also noticed the change, which opened up the topic for us.

"It's only natural to be more fluent and funny when you're not a zombie any more, no?" he asked.

Yes, I believe it is.

We began meeting every other week, and then every third. It was during one of those last meetings that Dave pressed the question "How does therapy work? Tell me the secret, because I really want to know how I got from there to here."

I had some thoughts on the subject, but I asked him to speak first. Dave claimed it was all me. Who else, he gushed, would have understood so much from his dreams, would have gleaned all I had from details like the tiny feet on his shirt, would have inspired him to persevere through the months he was feeling worse—and all this without the need for medication!

It's not false modesty to say that these were minor factors in his transformation. For every comment I made, someone else might have made ten more brilliant. Like all of us, Dave walked the earth hiding a great deal about himself in plain view. The anti-abortion shirt, after all, was one I had seen him wear many times before really noticing it. For that matter, I have often wondered what might have happened if, in our first session, I had taken seriously his wish to become more "communicable."

Dave Johnson changed because he took himself seriously, persevered in therapy even when it was making him feel worse, did some family research, and allowed himself to mourn. I fostered the pursuit of what he would eventually call the truth about himself. And I did that, above all, by setting a limit on our relationship. He tested the boundaries with me during the first few months by suggesting we meet as friends. Our work gained traction when I gently but unambiguously declined. Observing what happens in a session immediately following such an intervention often indicates its effect. It was in the very next meeting that Dave recounted the first dream he brought to therapy, the dream in which his father was neither dead nor alive. It felt to me as though he were saying, "If I can't seduce you, and you really are capable of being my therapist, then perhaps I can take the risk of being your patient."

"Can you promise me," Dave asked, "that my kids won't inherit this whole mess, that they won't go through the same stuff?"

I could more easily promise the opposite. Any Johnson children to come, I said, would most certainly struggle with intimacy, fidelity, love, and aggression. They, too, would need to make sense of themselves one day in light of the family's history, including: a philandering great-grandfather, a depressed and closeted grandfather, and a father whose immaturity led him to sire a child before he was ready to care for one. That said, I did feel that the next generation would hold certain advantages.

"You didn't start to feel you knew your dad until fifteen years after he died. You have the chance to break the mold by refusing to live 'upstairs' in silence."

"Talking helps because it leads to more talking," offered Dave.

"Um, yeah."

I wished I had said it myself.

•   •   •

"You know what I like about you, Deborah? You know what I appreciate? That we could agree to disagree about abortion."

"You were afraid I would try to change your mind."

"And you didn't. I mean, you made me think, but not like: 'You asshole, don't you see the error of your ways?' And I know this is a big cause of yours, or I imagine it is."

"Tell me what you imagine."

"That you're gung-ho."

"About being pro-choice?"

"Yeah."

"Can you say more?"

"It's not that I see you jumping up and down in the streets or anything. I figure you're the type to write to your congressman, or write articles. The things therapists do when they're gung-ho."

"It sounds like you have the impression that therapists keep their politics indoors."

"I guess. Am I way off base here? You're such a reserved person, I can't picture you going to rallies. Do you?"

I was going to be uncomfortable whether I answered directly or didn't.

"Actually, lots of therapists attend demonstrations. Me included."

"Oh yeah?" And then he looked at me, pinching his nostrils a few times while a thought as vexing as a Sphinx's riddle grew in his head. Dave said:

"You live in Philadelphia, don't you?"

"I do, actually."

Since Dave's therapy started, I hadn't seen him in front of the clinic. In fact, there had been a lull in anti-clinic activity at that particular site.

"I haven't been to a demonstration in a while," he volunteered. "It's really not my kind of thing, to tell the truth. Dr. Luepnitz, were we at the same demonstrations?"

Dave was able to pinpoint exactly when he had done his clinic duty. I knew that I had also been there on at least one of those occasions. So we had attended the same demonstration at least one time.

Dave wanted to know, of course, if I had realized this all along. I explained that we were well into the treatment before it occurred to me as a possibility. And in trying to place a face I had seen briefly in a large crowd, how could I be sure? The question of whether or not we'd been on opposite sides of the street didn't seem as important to me as the work we were able to engage together.

"Do you disagree?" I asked. "Do you wish I had brought it up the second it came to my mind?"

"I don't know. No. It's just weird. What if we had run into each other some day on the opposite side of the street?"

"We would have talked about it in the next session."

Therapists and patients should not be friends, but they usually do inhabit the same geographical region, and sometimes the same neighborhood. It's not unusual to run into one's therapist at some point at the bakery or at the movies. A colleague of mine was sitting with her husband in the waiting room of a fertility clinic when one of her therapy patients walked in with his wife. The four of them tried to greet each other respectfully while clutching small vials of body fluids.

Should psychotherapists avoid fertility clinics, movie houses, bakeries, and political demonstrations in order to avoid potential meetings with patients? Should patients screen therapists according to their most frequented venues? ("How many years have you been practicing, Doctor, and approximately how much time do you spend at the White Dog Café?")

It can't be done.

As awkward as such outside meetings can be, they do not have to wreck or derail the treatment, and can even be a boon. When a patient says she saw me walk into a restaurant with a man, I ask to know what she imagined. Here are some things I have heard in response to just such sightings over a period of several years, the man being the same:

- "I could tell from the way you were talking that he was your husband, but he didn't look at all like what I'd expected."
- "I'm a little embarrassed, because I could tell from the way you were talking that you weren't married, and I sort of wondered if he was your secret lover."
- "I was confused. I've always assumed you were a lesbian, so what were you doing dressed up on a Saturday night, with a man? I figured he was gay, too, and you had just come back from a conference or something."

Such fantasies can be explored, as they inevitably say more about the imaginer than the imagined. What would incline a patient to think of a therapist as "cheating," or gay, or married? What wish, fear, or identification is being addressed, and why at that moment in the treatment? The only thing to be avoided is the creation of a taboo subject. When a therapist or patient feels "something awkward happened between us, but we never could find a way to bring it up"—only then has something gone awry.

Dave continued: "You've been helping *me*—someone from the other side. When I told you that, didn't you want to kick my butt out the door?"

"No."

True statement. Only once in twenty-five years have I had to turn a patient away due to disparate political commitments. The difference in that case was so extreme that I knew I could not be of help.

"Did you decide *when* we would talk about this stuff?"

"I knew we would get around to it," I said. "And we can continue to talk about it in future sessions, if you like."

And, in fact, we did.

•   •   •

In *The Political Psyche*, British psychotherapist Andrew Samuels describes the results of a questionnaire he sent to practitioners around the world. Analysts acknowledged discussing a number of political topics in the consulting room, and the topics varied by nation. Americans were most likely to discuss gender politics in session; Israelis, Mideast events; and Germans, the environment.

This should be shocking only to those naive enough to insist that psychoanalysis and psychotherapy are somehow value-neutral activities perched somewhere above the world and politics. The fact is that our very theories of human development and therapeutic change are themselves political. As soon as we begin sorting out behaviors that are "pathological," "crazy," or "immature," we are revealing parts of a worldview. The Oedi-pus complex—as discussed by Freud and Rank in terms of a mother, father, and child—is considered by some to be politi-cally problematic. Given the fact that, at most, only half of American families conform to that model, insisting on its terms may be a way of denying the realities of social change. Many therapists over the past fifty years have argued for retain-ing the Oedipus myth in psychoanalysis but interpreting it in the broadest possible terms. Others have recommended throwing out the Oedipus complex entirely, insisting that it merely reproduces the violent and rivalrous relationships it aims to describe.

Certainly, new theories and new readings of old theories will be essential in the creation of a different kind of masculinity—one that would make Don Juanism less inevitable.

·   ·   ·

On the evening of our final session, Dave came in with an armful of flowers—peach, yellow, and red.

"Glads," he said, "because I'm very glad. . . . "

I was, too.

Dave sent holiday cards for a number of years. Three years after leaving therapy, he married Sylvie. They have a son.

4   A DARWINIAN FINCH

What a trifling difference must often determine which shall survive and which perish!
—Charles Darwin,
letter to Asa Gray

FOR MONTHS the professor had awakened to the same vague misery at four o'clock each morning—too early to rise, too late for a sleeping pill. There was nothing to do at that rude hour but cry, or stave off tears with ruminations: about her job, her life, archaic words for pain. Old English, she told me, had a special word—*uhtceara*—for the sadness or grief one feels in the hour before dawn.

Professor Pearl Quincey scheduled and then canceled several appointments with me. Each time we talked, she was "too fiendishly busy" or "too fiercely independent" for therapy. Each time, I learned a bit more of her story.

She was born in a shantytown in Jamaica and emigrated to the United States with her family as a young child. At fourteen, Pearl returned to the island to live with a schoolteacher aunt. A stellar student, she imagined herself teaching high school one day in Jamaica or in the American South. At a state college, Pearl's brilliance caught the attention of professors who urged her to aim higher. She had the potential to become a scholar, teach in a university, shine a light for other young people.

After an exhausting twelve years in graduate school—she was working to support her family back home at the same time—Pearl landed a position in an English department of no small reputation. The job offer, she said, was her life's proudest moment—and her family's as well. The little girl born in a hand-built house without hot water, the girl who'd been spat on by the children of her white teachers, was now an assistant professor of literature.

One year into her new life, however, it was clear something had gone terribly wrong. In the august university environment that appeared to offer everything, Pearl felt less stimulated, more isolated and depleted than ever before. Not even the death of her epileptic sister had left her feeling so hollowed out. Neither the strain of living with an overbearing stepfather nor the pain of watching a brother go to jail—nothing had quite prepared her for the loneliness of life in elite academia.

Where Pearl had imagined a convivial group of scholars devoted to students and involved with the community, she found small-minded cynics fighting over office space. Students complained of never having spoken to a professor. And as the only woman of color in the department, Pearl felt everyone taking her measure. Secretaries looked right through her; security guards followed her around the bookstore.

What was she doing in this wretched place? The answer: trying her best to get tenure—a job for life. The irony was not lost on her.

"Apparently I want the chance to become permanently— not just provisionally—miserable."

Pearl vowed to remain philosophical as her tenure vote came up. If she lost her first bid, no matter. She had been jumping through hoops for years; she would just keep jumping.

On the day the department actually voted her down, however, Pearl was devastated. Leaving the house the next morning, she drove the wrong way down a one-way street and stopped nose-to-nose with an eighteen-wheel truck, its horns blaring. The following day, she was awakened by a fierce attack of sciatica. The pain was so disabling she could barely get to the bathroom.

Ultimately, a sense of being robbed of her body, of being split into pieces, of actually not wanting to go on, became more frightening than the idea of seeking help. Pearl resolved to see me as soon as she could drive again.

I was pleased finally to meet her.

Pearl Quincey was a tall woman—six feet, perhaps—dressed in an aquamarine shift with a headwrap to match. Her skin was the color of English toffee, her voice a sturdy roux of West Indian and American inflections.

"I have shipwrecked," she said, accenting the second syllable. "I have washed up on your shore after all. Please forgive my false alarms."

I offered whatever combination of chairs and footrests might make her comfortable.

"I'm fine, actually, as long as I don't breathe."

Sitting across from Pearl, I myself had the sensation of holding my breath. This served as a first clue to my countertransference. I was identifying with her, mirroring her tight posture. On the surface, Pearl was an unlikely double for me, a medium-sized midwesterner. Nonetheless, I felt kinship. I have never fought a tenure battle, but I had beaten my head against enough institutional walls to imagine her weariness. My parents had not faced the indignities of racism or immigration, but they spent their lives doing hard physical labor, and like Pearl, I was the first in my family to get a formal education. Finally, like Pearl, I once overvalued self-reliance and shrank from the thought of confiding in strangers. Matching my breathing to hers alerted me to these runnels of thought. Empathy has its place in psychotherapy, but overidentification spells trouble, for each patient must be known on her own terms.

Professor Quincey leaned forward on the palms of her hands and said that the great frustration of the moment was not being able to read the titles on my bookshelves. No sooner had she made us smile than she began a full-bodied sob. Pearl was terribly ashamed of feeling bad. I asked why.

"I come from a line of strong women, and I have never broken down. I can't recognize myself in the fragile mess you see before you. And to fall apart over such petty stuff. It's mortifying. Have you ever known *anyone* this unraveled over *tenure?*"

Mentally, I composed a short list.

The "publish or perish" system and the factionalism of the academy unnerve many tenure candidates. Even that entitled white man Henry Kissinger claimed he left academic life because he "couldn't stand the politics."

The English department acknowledged Pearl's fine teaching and writing. However, they wanted to see more writing and less fine teaching. The idea of shortchanging students in order to crank out publications offended Pearl. But to leave the university—and disappoint her family, supporters, and students—was unthinkable.

When I suggested that we explore her hopes and misgivings about coming to see me, Pearl said:

"My mother is my closest confidante. In therapy, one delves into the family to pick it apart, and that would not be helpful to me. I need you to help me with the present, not the past."

I nodded. Because Pearl had mentioned isolation and loneliness, I asked about the people she counted on for support in the present. Did she have a spouse or partner? *No.* Children? *No way.* Pearl said she could see where my questions were headed, and

she decided to help me out. She had never been married or part-
nered, she said, and she did not see romance on the horizon.

"I don't date," said Pearl. "I've decided I'm not dateable."

"Not dateable?"

"I am a Darwinian finch," she said, shifting her long limbs
to the other side of the footrest. "Do you, by any chance, remember reading about the finches in *The Origin of Species?*"

"The ones who gave Darwin the idea of natural selection?"

"Exactly. Well, I am like a finch that has flown its little niche
for a new one. I've adapted in certain ways but I am, nonetheless, slightly different from the other birds, and now none can
recognize me as a potential mate."

I was surprised that this lovely, accomplished, thirty-four-
year-old woman had never had a serious relationship.

As for Darwin's finches, I had read about them in college—
who hadn't?—but I couldn't bring to mind the details of their
mating patterns. Pearl was using finch problems as a metaphor
for the problems of human beings who leave one social niche
for another. She felt different, unrecognizable in her current
environment. I wanted to know more about her migrations,
more about her original niche as well, but she had warned me
off with "That would not be helpful. . . ."

I have spoken before about the "yes" and the "no" alive in
every person who seeks therapy. Listening to Pearl I heard the
following: Yes, I would like to confide in you. No, that would displace my loyal family. Yes, I want to get help. No, that would
prove I needed it. Yes, I want to change my life. No, I don't. All
the things I do and everything I am have taken me this far.

"Don't get me wrong," said Pearl. "I'm not *unlovable*. I have
wonderful friends at home and in Jamaica."

"Would I be right in assuming that you're the person on
whom everyone depends for strength?"

Yes, she said. Her childhood nickname was "little Mama." Even her professors looked to her for wisdom, it seemed. Her brothers and sister had straightened out over the years, but their jobs were minimum wage. When her nephews' Catholic school bills came, when her mother needed a new roof, Pearl was called. That was another reason she could not give up her current job. The salary allowed her to help them.

I asked Pearl what she did to take care of herself when she was feeling bad. The answer: She organized a conference, taught Sunday school, or practiced calligraphy. Her list of a year's activities exceeded what most people take on in five. The term going through my head was one coined by the British psychoanalyst Melanie Klein: *the manic defense*. It refers to the flurry of activity some people use to mask even serious depression. It can work for years, and often is interrupted only by illness, exhaustion, or an accident. It occurred to me even as we spoke that this recent round of catastrophes might be the best thing that could happen to Pearl. Perhaps only this failure of an overdeveloped sense of duty would bring balance.

Shifting again on the couch, Pearl squeezed her back with both hands and asked if there were some way to think about psychotherapy that wasn't so "self-indulgent."

Perhaps because she had described herself as a finch, the idea of flying came to mind. When traveling by air, I reminded her, flight attendants advise adults to don their own oxygen masks before helping others. The moment I said it, I regretted the triteness of the analogy, but Pearl didn't seem to mind.

"You're talking about necessary selfishness, about first things first. OK. But how do you see the goals of this work?"

She imagined I would always be on the side of individual happiness, and not that of any larger purpose. There were days, she said, when she felt exactly the same way.

"Yesterday I considered telling the chairman that I would simply prefer not to get tenure, and I would just go home and teach third grade, or raise chickens and pigs."

"That's how you're feeling now? That you'd like to leave this whole mess behind?"

At this, Pearl started to cry into her fists, and after some time replied:

"No. Today, I want to say to you, 'I want tenure. Please help me keep my job.'"

Pearl had assumed my hopes for her would lie in a certain direction. I was glad she was able to articulate this assumption. Every practitioner must resist the temptation to steer the patient's course. Certainly it would give me pleasure to help Pearl break the glass ceiling, but who could say that that should be the goal of our work? Pearl herself vacillated from day to day about staying or leaving. My response was that our work could help her to clarify and implement her desire. That seemed to sit well with her.

In the meantime, what was her intention? To interview other therapists? To come back? She would come back, she said. The books, the feeling in the room, made her sense that good things had happened here. She made an appointment for the following week.

Pearl had positioned me in opposition to her family, at least to some degree. In her mind, I wanted to "pick apart" her family, and she was not about to do that. As for my identification with her, perhaps it was a way of bypassing our differences. There was, after all, no real comparison in our social origins. Maybe my inclination to merge our experiences reflected something about Pearl's relationship with her mother, her "closest confidante." All I knew about their relationship were the few things she had said in passing: they spoke on the phone each day, and both suffered from chronic back pain.

Uppermost for me was the matter of Pearl's engaging her dependency needs. In the past few decades, feminists have pointed out how difficult it can be for women, especially those who have taken on parental roles as children, to be helped instead of helping. A longing for succor can be masked in a hundred ways. I hoped Pearl would someday be able to lean on others, starting with me.

Finally, I was intrigued by her calling herself a "Darwinian finch." She had changed her name from a precious gem to a lonely bird, from the nickname "little Mama" to the name of a creature who would not mate. I turned to the bookcase to scan *The Origin of Species* before my next patient arrived. There, in between Darwin's *The Descent of Man* and Dickens' *Bleak House*, I found a telltale gap. A borrower had failed to return the book. I could not remember who it was, but I was fighting mad at the miscreant.

· · ·

Pearl showed up for her next appointment saying she had had two nights of restful sleep. She felt and indeed looked somewhat better. She could move her head freely, and had a fuller view of my consulting room and the books. I asked if anything caught her eye.

"There is a lot of psychoanalysis, of course. And feminism. . . . Hey now! You have good taste!"

"I do?"

"*Annie John*! Now there is a book a woman wants to see on her analyst's bookshelf."

We smiled at each other complicitly. I, too, loved Jamaica Kincaid's novel about a girl growing up in Antigua. So long did Pearl's gaze linger on that slender volume that I asked to hear her thoughts.

"The book is about—but you know the book is about a mother-daughter relationship. The sentence coming to my mind is so peripheral, I feel almost silly. . . . "

It was a good moment to introduce the "fundamental rule" of psychoanalysis: Say whatever comes to mind, no matter how important or irrelevant it may appear, no matter how pleasurable or unpleasurable.

In the passage she recalled, Annie John, age nine, is asked to read aloud in class. The sentence was: "The sound of my own voice had always been a calming potion to me."

I had only to smile.

"Heavenly stars, of course it's relevant! It's about talking, about the relief of speaking in front of the other, of being heard. I did feel better after our last meeting. I was surprised."

Jamaica Kincaid writes about the trauma of a daughter gaining independence from a mother and father in a normal family, a loving family. Little Annie gets up to read an original composition to the teacher. The composition describes the day a child is separated from her mother at the beach. She panics, and when they are reunited, the mother says, "I will never leave you." The teacher praises the story and adds it to the collection in the school library.

I knew that Pearl had left her mother at one point to live with her aunt. I was curious about that move and what it had meant to all involved. Had the transition been fluid, relatively free of conflict, motivated solely by the aunt's ability to provide better schooling? What role had Pearl's stepfather played? Had there been jealous tension among the adults, or furious rivalry among the siblings? How many kids were in this family, anyway?

Once again, I invited Pearl to talk. She could start anywhere.

"Well, in the English department. . . . "

Pearl resumed her tales of work, describing a radio program she had done with four other faculty members. The moderator had referred to the participants as Dr. Collins, Dr. Riley, Dr. Rossi, Dr. Levine, and *Pearl*. Absurdly, the topic of the program involved race and gender in academia.

"I felt anger beating drums in my ears each time someone called me by my first name. A part of me knew better than to call attention to it, but midway I heard myself saying aloud: 'Just a minute! Why are the others being called by their title, while I am "Pearl"?'"

"What happened?"

"The bemused host vowed to begin calling me 'Professor,' whereupon the four men sniffed—*almost* in unison: 'Personally, I'm not hung up on titles. Go ahead, and call me *John, George, Sneezy, Grumpy*.' Do you think I'm crazy to care about this? It's 1990, for the love of God!"

"Do I think *you're* crazy?"

Pearl didn't pause to hear supportive words from me. She had two other stories to tell. As I listened, I was aware of being enraged on her behalf and wanting to defend her. In fantasy, I landed on the scene, demanding to know why her colleagues did not understand that forgoing recognition of status was a luxury of the recognized.

Pearl was as much storyteller as analysand at that moment in the treatment. Any attempt on my part to intervene she gently deflected. Winnicott would say that she experienced my efforts as *impingements*, referring to the kind of parental attention that is felt by the child as usurping her nascent self. Years later Pearl would say to me, "I have been thinking about how few people in history have been listened to." Pearl needed me to listen.

A few weeks later, Pearl raised a complaint about the English department's self-described feminists. She saw them as posers, "purveyors of fried air." Nothing was "subversive" enough for them.

"In the meantime, these sisters wouldn't know a political thought if it stood up in their soup."

Valid as her critique might be, I had to wonder about its meaning in the transference. Although Pearl was cooperative in therapy, I felt that she was distant, still wary of me. Was it easier to critique the white feminists in her department than the white feminist sitting across from her in the room?

Pearl insisted that I was completely different from those women.

"No comparison," she assured me. "Apples and oranges. Chalk and cheese."

I was, she said, more like the women in her family.

"Really?"

I asked Pearl to explain and she said she would, but she was keen to tell me something else first. A program she had organized for Black History Month had been written up in the local newspaper. There was a department meeting on the day it appeared, and Pearl was sure that the chair would mention it. But no one said a word.

Pearl had decided not to get angry in those meetings any more. She was determined to be equable and patient in her dealings with colleagues. Nothing really worked, however.

Regardless of the tack Pearl took, those meetings had this in common: They left her feeling invisible, mocked, sometimes sick with self-criticism for days. I had to quiz her to find out that occasionally she did get compliments from colleagues. Those affirmations she managed to dismiss as disingenuous. For Pearl there were only two kinds of feedback: bad and insincere. As I listened to her, I began to hear the longing beneath her anger and frustration. It was fine, I said, to use

therapy to consider and reconsider strategy, and to vent her
rage. It was also important to address the longing for recognition. Pearl was less than smitten with this notion.

"Not because you're wrong, but because I don't fancy the
idea of needing validation from others. Remember, I'm usually
the one who ladles it out."

Precisely.

A vast amount of modern psychoanalytic theory deals with
our desire for recognition from other human beings. Since
Freud, no issue has so dominated the conversation about psychoanalytic theory or practice. Self psychologists, following
Heinz Kohut, write about the "mirror hungry" personality.
Students of Winnicott define the "good-enough mother"
largely in terms of her ability to *recognize* her infant. That means
seeing the child as a separate being, not simply an extension of
herself. Followers of Jacques Lacan believe that the ego is developed in the "mirror phase," which begins around eighteen
months of age. Lacanians emphasize the trouble caused by a
lifetime of searching for ourselves in a place external to us (either the physical mirror or the approving gaze of others). No
one else can tell us who we "really are." Even the physical object we call a mirror deceives by reversing right and left.

Feminist analysts have pointed out the politics of mirroring,
following Virginia Woolf, who famously remarked on women's
"delicious power of reflecting the figure of man at twice its
natural size."

We spend our energies figuring out whose recognition
counts—which mirror to consult and how to read the images
we discover. Some people are drawn to trick mirrors. They will
check their reflection only in the gaze of someone guaranteed
to diminish them. In contrast, a few lucky souls walk right by
mirrors that elongate flaws and foreshorten virtues.

Being the only woman or the only member of a racial minority at the workplace can make it much more difficult to be recognized and to believe in the recognition one finds. Minority status doesn't create the psychological need for recognition: it complicates it.

Early experience is influential if not determinative of our ability to see and be seen by others. Those who have not been recognized by parents don't know what recognition means, don't know quite how to seek it—and may be confused when it comes their way. I was, of course, interested in Pearl's experiences in her family. She let me know she had experienced "zero" recognition from her stepfather, but that she had been "loved and adored" by her mother and "deeply understood" by her aunt. We agreed that she needed to learn to accept recognition from people outside the family and particularly, it seemed, from male colleagues. I believed, moreover, that there were aspects of Pearl—her sexuality and desirability, for example— that had yet to be reflected convincingly by anyone.

It was in this session that I asked Pearl if she felt recognized by me.

"I do. To a surprising degree."

Would she let me know if I got her wrong?

That would be difficult, she admitted, but she would try to be candid.

In the meantime, Pearl needed to get back to work. There were no guarantees when it came to tenure, but the advice coming her way was to write. Pearl had plenty of ideas, but she was so anxious that the words would not come. She sat at her desk, night after nauseous night, still afraid of falling under the wheels of her depression, of getting caught in its gears. Pearl found herself counting the days between our weekly sessions.

"I'm a little annoyed," she said. "This is what I was afraid of. Therapy creates dependency."

I told her she was right, but that the dependency is of a particular kind—a temporary one. She was free to lean on our relationship as long as she needed it, but our goal was to set a date at some point to say good-bye. I asked what she was thinking.

"I don't know about the good-bye part, but the rest is comforting. You can be almost as comforting as my mother. I used to say my mother would have made a great lawyer, but now I think she should have been a therapist. I mailed her a photo of me taken at the department party, and she said the chairman looked like 'a snake in a suit.' When I told her the latest thing he had said to me, she just paused and said, 'Pearl Quincey, why are you so bothered by this heartless nonsense?' I wanted to crawl up in her lap, all six feet of me."

Comparing me with her mother was surely a compliment, although I could not compete with that lap!

"My mother would get these big knots in her shoulders and neck from scrubbing and lifting, so I would knead her back and then sit in her lap and rub her wrists."

They had been comforting each other for a long time.

Pearl was reminded once again of Jamaica Kincaid's novel:

"Annie John loves her mother's embrace, and says, '*It was in such a paradise that I lived.*' Well, that was me, too. That was us."

I asked Pearl if she wanted to elaborate, and it was at that point, three months into our work, that she began to describe the love story between her mother and her. It did not end when she moved in with her aunt. The two women in her life presented strong arms that reached the thousand miles from northern Florida to Kingston, the island's capital.

"I have traveled a fair amount, and although my mother claims to be interested in traveling, I can't get her to leave home. She has always said, 'I would rather see the world through your eyes.'"

"You have brought the world to your mother."

"When you put it like that, I understand why I'm so tired!"

Pearl felt that it was the least she could do, however. There was no one on earth she admired more.

"My mother has been my hero since I heard her talk back to the sheriff who came for my brother. Before that, even. She has been my hero since Haley's Department Store."

I asked if she would let me in on those episodes from childhood.

"Haley's was the famous Easter hat crisis. My mother made all our clothes, you see, and not many of those after my stepfather lost his job. Then he worked again for a while, and to make a long story short, we were visiting the city and allowed to buy Easter hats. I am in the fifth grade. Can you imagine what the inside of a department store looks like to me? I am on Cloud Nine looking at the pink and yellow chiffon flowers, thinking this work of art is going to be mine! But in twenty minutes it becomes clear that the clerks are not waiting on us. My mother tries nicely to get their attention, but there we stand while they wait on every white woman and girl in the world. Finally, a woman with hair that looks stiff like a lampshade turns to us. When mother points to the two pink hats, the woman balls up some greasy old tissue and puts it in the lining of the hats. Why? So our hair won't touch the white folks' merchandise! Tell me, what is the thing to do in that situation! My mother tries the hat on, but slowly, making everyone wait. And then, when the lady says, 'Make up your mind, poky, or get along!' she says, looking into the mirror the whole time: 'Madame, can't you see I have made up my mind? I have made up my mind to be treated like everyone else at this counter.' I was so proud of her!"

I could see little Pearl, nervous but thrilled to know *"this is my mother!"*

"Oh, Deborah, how we laughed about that woman! If you could have seen her face! The thing about Rita Quincey is that she's not bitter. To this day, she'll say: 'Those were the *times* we was living in.' When I tell her things that go on now at the college—that's what she can't understand. 'Educated folks with bad manners?' She can't quite fathom it."

Pearl adored her mother, and who wouldn't adore a mother like that? I could almost hear them talking on the phone at night in low tones, mocking the English department oddballs, giggling.

"I was twenty-one when my stepfather died, and my mother seemed to come alive in some ways—we all did. And yet she is still down there cleaning houses, won't travel. . . . "

Pearl interrupted her own shambling narrative to say I would be disappointed if I were looking for family scandals or abuse.

I said I wasn't looking for scandals; I simply wanted to know more about her early world. Now that she had clued me in a bit, how did she feel?

Pearl did not want her family "pathologized." She had heard social workers speak disparagingly about black families without any sensitivity to the strength of black families. There was nothing strange or unhealthy about her having lived with her aunt, she said. At times she had called them both "Mom," but that did not mean she was confused about who her mother was.

Pearl asked point-blank if I could see why she considered her mother her best friend. I could. She sounded irresistible.

Pearl waved her long amber beads playfully in my direction. She was glad I was getting the picture. She had been afraid, she said, that I would want to take her mother away from her.

•   •   •

Two weeks later Pearl remarked that while I knew a lot about her, she knew nothing about me. When I asked what she might like to know, her answer came back quickly. It was actually a relief, she said, not to know about my life, for if she did, she might worry and want to take care of me. Still, she was curious. . . .

Pearl's thinking is typical of psychotherapy patients. We feel curious about the therapist's life, but we don't really want our questions answered. I suggested that Pearl make a habit of stating her questions about me with the understanding that the questions need not be answered. The patient's fantasies are always more instructive than the facts.

Pearl saw me as someone who had undergone some great difficulty in life. And she guessed I had been widowed or divorced.

In the transference, I was becoming the good, slightly idealized mother. Like her mother, I was single and hardworking (Pearl was concerned about my long hours) and self-sacrificing (she guessed I did not take dinner breaks).

One evening when I happened to be thinking about her, Pearl telephoned. Very apologetically, she asked to run a work problem by me. Within ten minutes, she had outlined and solved her own problem, and I had only to listen and marvel at the fact that she had allowed herself the "indulgence" of calling. She said that if I hadn't picked up on the first ring, she might have lost her nerve. "You answered the phone because you knew I needed you tonight."

During this long moment in our work, Pearl Quincey could make me feel preternaturally attuned, effortlessly healing. Even when I did something that might have annoyed her, such as being late or saying "See you Tuesday" instead of Monday, she turned my foible to virtue. "You're just showing me that you, too, are human."

It was in such a paradise that we lived.

• • •

Pearl came in one afternoon several weeks later, talking about a good class. A male student had spouted off about the women's movement, insisting that there was nothing in nature more powerful than the maternal instinct, and the students had engaged each other in high-volume debate. During the next class, Pearl made a single and effective intervention: She read a passage from Darwin about instincts in animals that are more powerful than the maternal. The students buzzed in amazement. Pearl said that teaching had become a pleasure again now that she was feeling better.

I was distracted by this second reference to Charles Darwin.

"Pearl! Darwin again!"

"Again? Yes, the finches!"

Had I done my best to hunt those finches down? Finding that all four copies of *The Origin of Species* were checked out of the library, I had requested a "recall" but never followed up. I asked Pearl if she would refresh my memory about the finches and explain what they meant to her.

"Absolutely!" she said, and made a note to bring me the reference. At the moment, however, she had more pressing items for the session: a plan to get the tenure writing done, and a dream about writing with peacock-blue ink.

Pearl's view of dreams was different from mine. Whereas in the Freudian tradition I begin with the idea that the dream is a fulfillment of a wish, Pearl believed dreams had predictive power. The peacock-blue dream pleased her as it meant she would soon be "proud as a peacock" about her work.

"And why a *peacock?*"

"Why not?" she laughed.

•   •   •

The summer was approaching and Pearl had let me know early on that she would be interrupting therapy to spend time with her family in Florida. She had spent every summer of her life there and felt, indeed, that she belonged with the people who loved her most.

Pearl went a step farther than I expected. She said she was feeling so well that she was ready to stop therapy. She would come back in the fall to tie up loose ends, but she was grateful and pleased to be done. "I am feeling so much steadier. I feel like telling all my students that they should undergo psychotherapy."

I did my best to smile through this little speech, but I was nonplussed. Did she really feel she had "undergone psychotherapy"? I still knew relatively little of her history. Some patients offer more background information in two sessions than Pearl had in four months. And what about this business about being a finch, doomed to celibacy? Pearl had expressed candidly her fear of dependency, of course, and I had insisted on my intention to let her go. Now I felt like a Band-Aid she was peeling off. I suspected that she was detaching precisely because she was feeling close to me. I suggested that she might be talking of stopping therapy to avoid missing me over the summer. The notion did not ring true to her.

I asked if she didn't feel there were many more things for us to explore in therapy.

"Friends have nagged me for years about 'exploring' men. They cut out personal ads, tell me about dating services, leave their kids with me to babysit. Meanwhile, my mother is more forward-thinking than these big-city girls."

Rita Quincey had told her daughter long ago that women no longer needed to marry. Rita described a television show she had seen about the Delaney sisters, who credited their hundred and four–plus years to the fact that they never married. "We didn't have husbands driving us crazy," they had told reporters.

I asked Pearl if she thought my wanting to explore her personal life was a step toward marrying her off.

"Well, I don't know what you have in mind, and that's the point. Who decides when a person is healthy?"

Regarding the goals of therapy, Freud said simply: *lieben und arbeiten*, to love and to work. Wisely, he did not define either term. Others have not hesitated to do so, some with disastrous results. Melanie Klein wrote a paper on the requirements for the termination of analysis. Before adding her own contribution, Klein summarized what she considered to be the accepted and "well-known criteria" for termination, including "an established potency and heterosexuality." Given all he did to normalize homosexuality, this is not a criterion Freud would have accepted or recognized. Reading the case studies of certain British and American practitioners, one could easily get the impression that their goal was to help people adapt to middle-class social codes.

I had already devoted a good portion of my career to contesting this normative revision of Freud. It felt odd to be identified with the conservative view!

I find nothing suspect about a woman's choosing to live without marriage or children, but Pearl seemed not to have done any choosing. She had expressed neither conflict nor curiosity about romance or sex. I stated the obvious: There is no single definition of the good life. However, I argued, in this psychotherapy which she had elected to undergo, she had introduced an enigmatic statement about her identity. I suggested that before finishing our work, we get to know more about Pearl as "Darwinian finch."

She agreed.

I was pleased at Pearl's willingness to challenge me in this session and to let me push back. It showed her ability to move out of the idyllic mother-daughter harmony into something more complex. Perhaps it was just this complexity, this dissonance, that she dreaded, and she would rather leave therapy than face it.

The months that followed provided me with space to reflect on my Darwinian finch. Pearl had said there was something about her that was "slightly different," resulting in her not being recognized by men as desirable. I knew that she did not mean anything obvious like her height, which might have intimidated boys in school. Pearl had let me know she was talking about very subtle, "hardly visible" differences. The only other clue she had offered in passing was that academic men felt she was not quite like other academic women, and that men in her hometown found her "citified" and "strange."

Allowing for the complications caused by class migration, I couldn't readily account for the extreme nature of Pearl's situation. Why had she not found a single man in one of those places who would love her precisely for her differences, who would find her not odd but extraordinary?

Given the enormous number of girls who have suffered sexual trauma in their early lives, I had to wonder if she had been molested. Many abused girls say just that: that they feel

fundamentally "different" in some vague and painful way. Pearl
had warned me early on not to expect surprises or secrets. We
know, however, that many people repress traumatic events and
remember them later, sometimes with corroborating evidence
from the abusers or from hospital records.

I wondered also if the "unrecognizability" in question had
to do with sexual orientation. Was it possible that her desire
was for women, but that this had been less acceptable to her
than abstinence?

There was no evidence for my hypotheses either in the content of her sessions or in the transference. Some people who
have been abused are so imbued with the victim-victimizer dynamic that they continue unconsciously to re-create it everywhere. Sitting with Pearl, I never felt: "This woman is expecting
to be abused by me." Nor did I feel the opposite (also common):
"This person is expecting me to submit to her emotional abuse."

Before leaving on vacation, I finally put my hands on a copy
of *The Origin of Species* in order to read the chapter on finches.
To my everlasting surprise, there was no such chapter! Not only
that, but the book indexed not a single entry for finches. I decided it had to be a bad index, and began reading the text from
the beginning. Pigeons, mockingbirds, and tortoises inhabited
those pages that changed the world, but no finches. Perhaps
Darwin described them in *The Descent of Man*, his book that explores natural selection in depth. Not a mention. Finally I found
a single paragraph about the Galapagos finches in *Diary of the
Voyage of the H.M.S. Beagle*—a book I had never read. That lesser
work was written in 1837. Why had the finches not made it into
his 1859 opus? And how had Pearl and I come to believe we
had read a nonexistent passage? It was an extraordinary *folie à
deux*, I thought, and yet something I could not discuss with my
partner in illusion, precisely because she had flown home.

As the August air chilled to a fall breeze, I was pleased to see Pearl's name in my appointment book once again.

She walked into my office looking relaxed, sporting beaded plaits, and carrying a copy of *The Origin of Species*. Pearl said she had had a wonderful summer.

"But I have strange news for you. Someone stole a chapter out of this book," she said.

I knew what she meant.

"Well, I have some library work cut out for me," she said.

"Pearl, tell me what you remember about the finches."

She drew a deep breath, and finally embarked on her explanation. Pearl informed me that Charles Darwin had started off his voyage believing in the fixity of species. In the Galapagos Islands, however, he found thirteen distinct species of finches, one per island. He realized that their isolation from each other had allowed them to evolve into distinct species, not just varieties of the same species.

"But what does the story mean to you?"

"Some of those thirteen species look different from each other, but others are so much alike that the human eye can't distinguish them. Only the finches can. A bird who flies to a different area, despite sporting the same feathers and singing the same song, will be excluded on the basis of having a beak that is a hair's breadth different from the others."

"OK, so these birds, somehow—mysteriously to us—decide that a new bird on the block is just slightly different, and then deem that bird to be . . . "

"Undateable."

Pearl was more comfortable applying her intellect to the problem than moving close to her emotions. She had not spent much time thinking about why this particular story had resonated so deeply with her. She had, however, begun looking up everything she could find on the topic. There was a good deal of helpful material, and Pearl made copies for me with passages highlighted in yellow.

The key to our conundrum lay in an article written by historian of science Frank Sulloway. Pearl flew in one afternoon, waving it in the air.

"This article is called 'Darwin and His Finches: The Evolution of a Legend.' Are you ready for this?"

She was hardly seated on the couch when she began reading aloud to me:

> [F]ar from being crucial to his evolutionary argument, as the legend would have us believe, the finches were not even mentioned in *The Origin of Species*. . . . In spite of the legend's manifest contradictions with historical fact, it successfully holds sway today in the major textbooks of biology and ornithology, and is frequently encountered in the historical literature on Darwin. It has become, in fact, one of the most widely circulated legends in the history of the life sciences, ranking with the famous stories of Newton and the apple. (p. 40)

Pearl looked up at me. I was still standing, too amazed to move. The moment I sat down and made eye contact, we both burst out laughing.

"No, wait—there's more!" she said.

Darwin apparently did notice the finches, but collected relatively few. Having packed them together, he had trouble labeling them. Observing the finches didn't turn him into an evolutionist. Rather, it was his conversion the following year to evolutionary views that allowed him to look differently at those finches. It was a colleague—a man who, ironically, didn't believe in evolution—who had to tell him the finches were actually different species.

"So the legend romanticizes a messy bunch of events," I said, "removing the story of his dependence on other thinkers."

"Right. And apparently the serious work on the finches wasn't done until 1947, by a man named David Lack. It was he who observed that even the seemingly identical finches were careful not to interbreed."

Some scholars, we learned, believe they should be called "Lack's finches." The story does not end there, however. Evolution, as we now know, is not something that happened eons ago but something continuously operating. Later researchers found that under certain conditions, finches of different species do "date" and mate. Fully 10 percent of the finches on one of the Galapagos Islands are now hybrids. And the birds who have mated with those outside their group are the most robust of all!

Pearl was fascinated with the topic. The finch studies spoke to her like writing on the wall, and her excitement was contagious. Sketches of shiny black birds with impressive beaks, photocopies of data in infinite shades of gray, found a messy nest high on my old Ikea bookshelf.

The conclusion Pearl drew from her voluminous reading was that to be a Darwinian finch or a Lackian finch was by no means to be doomed to neglect and exclusion.

A source of ongoing dismay for Pearl was not being able to place the moment she had named herself a Darwinian finch. She remembered only writing a report in high school on Darwin, and finding him a sympathetic character—indeed, an intellectual hero.

This man whose ideas shook the world was a humble preacher who started out believing in the constancy of species. He allowed both observation and argument to change his mind. This was what a good scientist must do, she told her students. Or a good scholar.

Biographers have described Darwin as a homely man of mediocre intelligence, a bad speller, and an imperfect researcher who made terrible gaffes in sorting his specimens. He seemed to me an unlikely hero for Pearl, the elegant intellectual, meticulous in her work, possessed of a lapidary wit. Not odd at all, on second thought. One of the few things she had told me about her stepfather was that he had to be right all the time; there was no changing his mind. It occurred to me that Darwin had appeared at a moment in her young life as the flawed but gentle father for whom she longed.

Eventually, Pearl decided that regardless of where she had found the finch fable—updated with certain details—it stuck because she needed it to be true. "Mating" had for her an aura of impossibility, and it was more comfortable to think of this poetically as destiny rather than choice. What had become of beautiful Pearl, the woman trapped inside the story? Why not do some research on her own name?

On this subject of her name, Pearl had some things to tell me right then and there. Other facts she learned only later, after speaking with her mother.

She had always liked her first name, and remembered clearly the day her aunt showed her that precious pearls come in shades of black and white. And while she knew she had been named for her mother's mother, she had not known why.

"My mother had always told me that she didn't get along with her mother, who was crazy and beat her, but spared her sister, my aunt. My mother hoped that naming her pretty baby 'Pearl' would win her mother over."

Pearl had never liked her last name, "Quincey," because it belonged to the stepfather she despised. It might have been some slave's first name, a hundred fifty years back, she said. She had simply never wanted to know anything about him or his family.

I let Pearl know that I believed in asking questions about our names. She agreed in principle, but made it clear that it might take years before she would be ready.

The name "Pearl Quincey" contained worlds of meaning: the attempt of a daughter (Rita) to win over a "crazy" mother, the story of that daughter's rivalry with her favored sister, an association with beautiful jewels in black and white, and a connection to slavery with all its savage destruction of names and subjectivities.

While speaking to her mother about names, Pearl had been careful not to mention therapy. It was important that Mrs. Quincey not have to think of Pearl as anything but invincible. She had been disappointed to learn that "after all the trouble and fuss" Pearl still did not have tenure.

"But they will raise your salary, no?" her mother asked.

Pearl admitted to me for the first time that she felt pressure from her mother to succeed. She also told me that she had felt bad about studying literature, as her mother had wanted her to become a famous scientist or doctor and discover a cure for cancer. Who could blame this mother, whose life had been crushingly difficult, for wanting to live through her child? Of course the family wanted Pearl to become a big name. Pearl wanted it, too.

The uncovering of the finch myth marked a turning point in our work. Pearl said: "It would make any person say, 'What else do I assume to be true that is not?' It feels like an open door where one expected none."

I wondered how she felt about the fact that I, too, had believed in the myth of Darwin's finches.

"You did and you didn't," she said. "You kept asking me to talk about it, or I never would have done the research."

My asking questions about her name is something I owe to my interest in the work of Jacques Lacan. No analyst since Freud has so keenly appreciated our debt as human beings to language, to the register of the symbolic. Even before we speak, we are spoken about, says Lacan. Before we are loved and held by mothers and others, before birth, and sometimes years before our conception, we have already been the subject of talk. In some families, a male or female child has been long awaited—or dreaded. In others, a child may be conceived as a replacement for a lost baby or relative. Parents rich and poor, sick and well, imagine all manner of things for their children. These expectations—along with cultural conversations about the value of children, male and female, born in and out of wedlock to parents young and old, straight and gay—cannot fail to affect children's subjectivity, the way they will say "I am." Sometimes all a person knows about this complex history of being spoken about is his or her name and namesake. Names, given to us in a deceptively simple gesture, are stuffed with hope, memory, and fear.

Investigating the "stuff" of our names and our origins can provoke anxiety, but failing to do so often ends up the more perilous choice. For an example of such peril, we need go no farther in myth or literature than Sophocles' Oedipus. The name "Oedipus" means "swollen foot" and refers to his bio-logical father maiming him as an infant before having him abandoned in the woods. Oedipus is rescued by a herdsman and raised by adoptive parents. When, as an adult, Oedipus learns from the oracle that he will kill his father and marry his mother, he flees the adoptive parents, assuming the oracle meant them. Vainly trying to escape his fate, Oedipus of course fulfills it instead, killing his biological father and marry-ing his biological mother.

Oedipus showed exceptional cleverness in solving the riddle of the Sphinx. But he was neither clever nor curious enough to solve his own riddle, the riddle of his name. For Lacan, the Oedipus tale is not so much about the infamous family triangle as it is a case of mistaken identity. An aging Oedipus, blind and in exile, finally undertakes a kind of self-examination. Something we might call transformation or redemption comes as he acknowledges and accepts his wounded self. The formerly proud Oedipus addresses King Theseus poignantly at Colonus:

> *I come to give you something, and the gift*
> *Is my own beaten self; no feast for the eyes;*
> *Yet in me is a more lasting grace than beauty.*

Jacques Lacan understood the Oedipus complex in the lives of actual men and women, analogously. We are, each one of us, embarked on a mission involving mistaken identity. In order to connect with other people—in order to answer our own "Who am I?"—we use names, academic degrees, medical diagnoses, family prognostications, and social myths. I am a "poor little rich kid," "the daughter of alcoholics," "the overachiever," "the forgotten middle child," "a Darwinian finch." Many of us never question these—cannot stop taking them for granted—until we falter, break down in some way.

Pearl had entered therapy thinking about herself more confidently as a Darwinian finch than as, say, "Professor Quincey." One could argue, of course, that "Professor Quincey" is also a mistaken identity. Alone, it does not carry the truth about Pearl. For Lacan, all identities are mistaken in the sense that they are superficial, partial. We use them to function in the world, but we need always to remember the cost. The point is not to go nameless, to refuse the question "Who am I?", but to keep the conversation about identity going. This is the work of psychotherapy: to learn both to assume an identity and to call it into question. It is one of the principal ways that talking helps.

• • •

It was around this time, in the second year of her therapy, that Pearl began to speak about the rest of her family, and to tell more of her story:

"My mother got pregnant with me the first time she had sex, at fifteen, with a fourteen-year-old boy named Owen Platt. My aunt married a white man with enough means to help us leave Jamaica. In Florida, my mother met Derek Quincey, a dark-skinned, broad-shouldered man who married her for her looks. I believe she fancied him at first. He was older and seemed interested in providing for us. His father was killed in a fight over fifty cents lost in a card game. That's when his drinking went out of control."

Mr. Quincey beat his sons, and Pearl lived in terror of his mad fits.

When Pearl had the chance to live with her aunt, Derek opposed it, saying that "the Rasta bastard" would go wild there and start popping out babies. Her mother cited her studiousness and said they should let her go. Pearl choked on the thought of leaving her mother behind, but she wanted to escape her stepfather. When her brother broke his arm, a drunken Mr. Quincey—who had hated doctors since a white physician refused his mother care—knelt on the boy's chest, cursing and insisting he could set the bone. Seeing her mother helpless against his evil, Pearl felt hate for her, too. Pearl vowed to be victimized by no man.

The exception to Derek's no-doctor rule involved little Ellie, born with a seizure disorder. For Derek to favor—of all children—this sick and weak one! Pearl remembered feeling superior to Ellie because the little girl had much darker skin than hers. Pearl had never voiced her resentment of this child to anyone. Not a word.

I made sure to ask Pearl during these sessions how she felt talking about her family.

"I feel a twinge. When I started to talk—did you notice?—I sort of whispered like they might be in the next room listening. But you know, they aren't. This is my life, and these stories belong to me, and I want to tell them."

Pearl said she wanted to say a bit more before we stopped for the day.

As a teen-ager, she continued, boys did not approach her, and she was relieved. She would do anything before proving her stepfather right and getting sent home. Better to outdo the adults in the business of good behavior.

Many a high-school girl feels insecure or overlooked, of course. Pearl's awkward stage continued through college. She insisted she was not noticed by men—not by short or tall men, not by men who grew up in the South, North, the West Indies, or abroad. She did not feel ugly, just different. "It was like I wore a sign that said 'I don't do sex, marriage, or babies.'"

I liked this talk of wearing a sign. It suggested she realized that, far from being unrecognizable in some essential way, she had made choices. The "sign" had served her well. As a woman of color, she had always to be at the top of her class to prove that she was as good as the rest. Without financial resources and with a family to support, she had worked a couple of jobs at all times. Pearl had become one with her work. A man would have been a distraction.

I asked if she ever felt otherwise now—that a relationship could make life better.

Pearl looked away and shook her head. I had the feeling I was about to get a talking-to. She asked if I had any idea of the statistical odds against an educated black woman her age finding a suitable male partner. I let her know I understood that the demographic facts were not encouraging.

"Nonetheless, I'm asking you, Pearl: What if you did meet someone you liked? Would you be interested in a relationship?"

"If it were 'raining men'? Yes, but still, who would I find to put up with me? I'm not a youngster; I'm set in my ways."

"Keep talking."

"Who would have me? I'm a terrible cook. I don't want to take care of any more kids. . . . I mess up everyone's stereotype, don't you think? Is there a man anywhere looking for a tall, guileless black lady who reads a book a day and keeps nothing in the fridge but Popsicles?"

Her questions were beginning to change. In fact, during this period, I never knew what she would bring up.

Pearl walked into her next appointment asking, "How do you do it, Deborah?"

"How do I do what, Pearl?"

She wondered how I balanced work and social life, marriage, kids, romance, private time. She believed I held certain secrets, both the keys to her own mythology and the keys to living. Would I share them or keep them to myself? If she did meet someone, could she count on me for advice? What if she fell for someone I didn't like? Could I stand to hear the details of pursuit and courtship?

Pearl wanted reassurance that I could tolerate her becoming sexually active. Her parents had managed to foreclose her curiosity and experimentation. Pearl wanted to be sure I would not be put out, frightened, censorious, or jealous of her new adventures.

Three months into our work on these issues, Pearl had coffee one day with a psychology professor. This led to weeks of dating that felt sexually charged. She enjoyed the physical contact a lot, which she described as mostly "kissy-face" (accent on face).

When Pearl announced those events to me, I almost knocked over the small bowl of roses at my right. She had gone from coffee to her first kissy face in three dates? So matter-of-factly?

Only then did Pearl clarify: Although she had not done any formal dating in college, she had fancied certain boys, been flirted with, danced a lot. She had even had a bit of sexual experience in graduate school. It simply hadn't added up to anything, she said. Neither to love nor to hope.

With regard to her new psychologist friend, the challenge came in the time between dates, when she was waiting for him to call. She would feel needy and pathetic. How she missed being totally in control.

I let her know she did not sound pathetic by any means. The desire to be perfect, in total control, had become a motif, and I asked if she could say more about it. It was a desire she connected with her mother's love. She had lived to be her mother's perfect daughter, thereby vindicating Rita's life of sacrifice. Pearl was beginning to glimpse the error in this: There were no perfect daughters; and showing weakness, admitting to desire, were not decisions taken against her mother.

When the psychology professor returned to his former girlfriend, Pearl was very disappointed, but she did not regret the experience. She felt a spell was broken. Pearl seemed to me more relaxed and confident, less stern a taskmaster to herself.

She had even gone out and bought a used piano, not for her nieces and nephews but for herself!

I was shocked, therefore, on arriving home from a long weekend to find a crisis message from Pearl. Her sciatica was back; she was in grinding pain. It occurred just hours after receiving some news by mail. On the strength of four chapters, a major academic publisher had accepted her book, virtually ensuring her tenure.

Pearl told me about this on the phone. She knew she had every reason to celebrate, but she felt awful. Why had the good news triggered her symptom? Why should success be so closely paired with pain? When I asked Pearl for her thoughts, she recounted the nightmare she had had that morning.

I am sitting high up in a tree, enjoying the view. I can't believe I have climbed so high. I look below and see a creature drowning. It is part kitten, part rabbit or rat. I am horrified, and yet happy the thing is not mine. I woke up in a sweat.

I asked Pearl to say whatever came to mind about the dream.

"That's me up in the tree, looking down. And the creature, I think, has to be Ellie."

Here was another boat I had missed. It was during our very first conversation that Pearl had mentioned the sister who died. I assumed she died as a direct result of the epilepsy. It turned out, however, that she drowned in the creek near their house.

Pearl said that her brothers kept a canoe near the creek, and had been warned about keeping Ellie away from it. One day she wandered off just long enough to throw her toys inside and try to push it in the water. It's possible that she had a seizure before falling, because no one heard her cry out. They found her facedown in the water.

Fifteen-year-old Pearl was terrified that Derek would blame her for Ellie's death. He did. If Pearl had been home where she belonged, he said, the child would be alive. Pearl was torn between a desire to go back and comfort her mother and a wish to stay with her aunt and finish school. Her mother made the decision for her, insisting that Pearl's education was paramount. Pearl was ostensibly relieved, and no one guessed her guilt. Friends and family had gathered around the Quincey home to mourn the child's death. Pearl, meanwhile, was sitting in a girls' school studying algebra and French.

The dream made the conflict almost unbearably clear. Pearl had climbed higher than she had ever imagined, and loved the view. She had reached that point, however, only at the expense of her sister's life. "The thing was not mine" are the words she uses in the dream, connoting her envious disparagement of Ellie.

Pearl dealt with her embarrassment of riches in the way she knew how—by giving away all she could. Ellie's death, she said, redoubled the drive to justify her privileged position. No one would accuse her of living high on the hog. She would work harder and accept fewer rewards than anyone. It was no surprise that she could not feel joy about the prospect of success.

Pearl was not the first patient of mine to become depressed over good news. One astute man observed that the unconscious seems to put an "absolute value sign" on events. Thus, we are disrupted by big changes, be they in the positive or negative direction. People have committed suicide on both losing fortunes and winning them.

Throughout her second year of therapy, Pearl talked a lot about messages the family had given her about staying and leaving, about independence and family loyalty, about gratitude and self-indulgence. These can be complex knots for any family to untangle, but in those whose young members actually change social class, they seem particularly gnarled. Poor and working-class parents generally want their children to have opportunities they missed. Their children take up the mandate to succeed and, in so doing, end up in a world foreign to their parents. They not only do a different kind of work, they also eat different foods, enjoy different entertainment, and hold different political views. The young person in such a family may feel that, in order to show loyalty (through success), he or she must inevitably reject the family's traditions. And the young person may feel tremendous guilt about surpassing siblings and cousins economically. In some families, the successful member tries to convert those left behind to new tastes, as though envy might magically dissolve if everyone would just eat brioche and read the *New York Times* in their designer pajamas.

Pearl had tried her best to remain part of the clan. She permitted herself to enjoy certain fruits abroad, but only if she shipped some home. She was allowed to do well, but not to feel well. Giving up the dream of romantic love, she decided, was a kind of deal she had struck with God. He had taken her sister; she would soldier on, living and working for two. Loneliness would be the price she paid for her vertiginous luck.

Freud wrote evocatively about people he described as "wrecked by success." He found it bewildering, but true, ". . . that people occasionally fall ill precisely because a deeply rooted long-cherished wish has come to fulfillment. It seems then as though they could not endure their bliss." Freud gave several examples, among them that of a professor awarded a coveted university chair after the death of its occupant.

"He fell into a state of melancholy which unfitted him for all activity for some years after."

The problem, as Freud saw it, was that the immediate success in these cases resonated with a longed-for but taboo success from early life, namely the Oedipal desire to possess fully one parent, displacing the other. The feeling in adulthood that one has finally "done it" wraps certain people in the grip of a guilty wish long repressed.

There was, in Pearl's recent success, the revival of some elements of her family complexes. Pearl's underestimated rivalry with Ellie—her stepfather's favorite—had contributed, we concluded, to her years as a confirmed celibate. Her choice of the label "Darwinian finch" condensed an astonishing number of aspects of her identity. It meant that she bore the proud name of Charles Darwin, an influential scientist with a gentle soul. It meant that she was a bird, that is, a creature destined to migrate and therefore expected to leave home. Pearl would not mate or have children, thus escaping the humiliations her mother had known—living with a bully and a drunk, seeing her children abused, and giving up a life of her own.

There is another matter that comes into play in this conundrum known as "incomplete mourning" or "frozen grief." Sometimes we deal with a lost loved one by identifying unconsciously with that individual. In choosing to be a finch, Pearl was not only giving up part of her self, she was also becoming Ellie. Ellie had always been known as a child who would not grow up and have a full adult life. She wandered off one afternoon, dreaming of we-know-not-what, pushing and pulling at the little canoe she longed to board. She shipwrecked instead. Pearl had, too: indeed, this was the first thing she said about herself on entering my office. "I have shipwrecked. . . . washed up on your shore after all."

•   •   •

In the third year of therapy, Pearl met Joshua, a physician and native of Cameroon. Joshua listened and he talked. He loved his own work, and he enjoyed Pearl's passion for hers. He delighted in her beauty and talent, and he did not idealize her.

The finch was in love for the first time. Daily she endured the highs and lows. I was glad to support her in those dizzy moments. When she worried that she "did not deserve, . . ." I reminded her that she did deserve. When she asked if her mother could adjust to her being in love, I assured her we would continue to work on that.

As their relationship progressed toward sexual consummation, I found myself filled with delight for Pearl, and only slightly jittery. Had we talked enough about her fear of engulfment and of engulfing, her fears of penetration and of pregnancy, for her to accept the pleasures of sex?

Yes, apparently. Pearl grew to love her intimacy with Joshua. The most difficult part was her mourning over lost time.

"This whole world called the body," she said beautifully, "all these years could have been mine."

Pearl's plaits grew to shoulder length and the beads more ornate. Emboldened, fledged, no longer wary, she enjoyed everything she did in a heightened way.

Those floaty months of pleasure—how long can human beings bear them? Pearl was not sure how to tell Joshua she needed more time alone. At length they had "the talk," about time spent together and alone. This should have solved the problem, she thought. However, there were days she would have traded all the pleasures of love for a month alone to write and think. Sometimes she wished for no relationship at all.

"I'm ashamed. I must be the textbook definition of neurosis. Do you think I might be one of those people who simply have no talent for happiness?"

I did not. I thought she was smack in the middle of the porcupine dilemma. Whenever Joshua held back, she rushed toward him; when he made himself available, she withdrew. To me she was not an exotic bird, unchosen and unchoosable, but a porcupine like everybody else—a creature social and capable of reproducing, but one who would forever seek the right distance between the painful extremes of entanglement and isolation.

Pearl was eager for her mother to meet Joshua, but Rita came up with a dozen reasons why she couldn't do so. I wondered if this was about Joshua being a physician, or about his being African. "I think it's about his being a man," said Pearl. "It's about his being not her."

Pearl had always been glad not to have one of those mothers who were always needling their daughters to marry. She was unprepared, however, for what turned out to be a prolonged indifference—even hostility—on her mother's part toward her relationship. That her mother, always proud of her achievements, should not join in her delight over this development filled Pearl with anger.

Here we labored for a long time. It was, perhaps, the most profound piece of mourning Pearl had to face—less dramatic but infinitely more bitter than mourning her sister, or even "lost time."

Rita Quincey had wanted to spare her daughter the disappointments of marriage. No doubt she also felt protected by her unmarried daughter, and loved being Pearl's confidante. Despite her peregrinations, Pearl seemed to be the one child who would never leave her.

It was at this point in therapy that Pearl reconsidered an interpretation I had made years earlier: that the sciatica was yet another means of staying connected to her mother. The notion had been meaningless to her three years ago; it was simply a coincidence, she said, that both she and her mother suffered from chronic back trouble. Now she saw it differently. The pain they shared in this particular part of the body marked them both as women who did hard physical work. They could commiserate, they could feel for each other. As a teenager, Pearl realized, the pain had allowed her not to have to feel that she was a spoiled girl on permanent holiday. Like her mother, she was a hard-working black woman, laboring to support her family. A symptom that made her feel connected to her mother's body would not, she realized, be a symptom easily given up.

Much has been written about the mother-daughter relationship in the past few decades. Some of this writing refutes the rather dim view Freud took of the bond between mothers and their female children. In the tendency of mothers to overidentify with daughters in the early, "pre-Oedipal" stage, Freud saw the origins of women's "lesser capacities" for autonomy and objectivity. In the 1970s and 1980s psychoanalytic feminists wrote about mother-daughter identification in a more complex way. Indeed, they said, the blurred ego boundaries between a mother and her girls may lead her to assume she knows their feelings before they do. Yes, it may lead them to cling to each other. What is lost in terms of autonomy, however, may be made up in the positive qualities of empathy and loyalty.

The psychoanalyst Nancy Chodorow writes about differences between boys and girls at the pre-Oedipal stage. The boy's first intimate connection in life is with a cross-sex parent, and the girl's with a same-sex parent: in both cases, the mother. Boys are expected to switch their identification and become like the males in their family. Girls do not experience that rupture; they are expected to maintain their original identification.

Chodorow maintains that this fact contributes to girls' greater tendency for continuity and connection to others. It can also trap girls into those very things, however.

Therapists, fiction writers, and memoirists have set themselves to describing this set of issues. On the subject of mothers and daughters, Jamaica Kincaid is again most eloquent. In adolescence, Annie John reflects:

> Something I could not name just came over us, and suddenly I had never loved anyone so or hated anyone so. But to say hate—what did I mean by that? Before, if I hated someone I simply wished the person dead. But I couldn't wish my mother dead. If my mother died, what would become of me? I couldn't imagine my life without her. Worse than that, if my mother died, I would have to die, too, and even less than I could imagine my mother dead could I imagine myself dead.

Pearl was beginning to distinguish her desires from her mother's, as some girls do in adolescence. She wrote letters home, angry and plangent. She read drafts to me until she had the tone just right. Pearl never stopped loving her mother, but her capacity to love, admire, and desire expanded its embrace. Instead of phoning home for a few minutes each day, she began calling for an hour on Sundays. Pearl prevailed upon her brothers and sister to do some of their mother's banking and doctor's appointments—things she had done from a distance.

Pearl practiced some distancing moves on me. She, who had never canceled a session without a good reason—and certainly not without notice—was now canceling frequently. There were three occasions on which I would have charged her, in fact, had I followed my policy meticulously. I had explained the cancellation rule to her at the outset. When I raised the matter once again, Pearl refused to engage me, insisting that she had been "fiendishly busy" of late. I took that fact into account and fortified it with some vague sense of her specialness. The latter, I eventually realized, was something I needed to analyze in myself.

The words going through my mind were: "It's Pearl. How can I charge her when she . . . has had such a hard life . . . never believed in therapy in the first place . . . has done so well . . . is someone who sacrifices for others, and who wouldn't understand my need to charge for missed sessions?"

This was not trivial stuff! Many patients come in skeptical about therapy. Many have had hard lives. Pearl was by no means the most deprived person I had ever had in my care. What exactly was going on here?

I believe we were reenacting the relationship she had with her mother, in which clear boundaries were sacrificed and conflict foreclosed by the wish to be close and unique to the other. I had to ask myself if cultural factors were in play as well. How else to make sense of my musing that "she wouldn't understand my policy"? The more I thought about this particular free association, the more condescending and suspect it sounded. Was this a bit of unconscious racism dressed up as magnanimity? I half-hoped the issue would go away, but it did not. Pearl then called to cancel a session because she wasn't feeling well. We rescheduled the appointment but she didn't show up. She called that evening to say she had forgotten about it completely. I mentioned I would have to bill her for the missed session.

At the time of the phone call, Pearl hadn't protested, but in our next session, I noticed her fighting tears as she wrote out the check. I encouraged her to speak.

Therapy was an extravagance in the first place, she said. To pay this hefty sum for no session at all was outrageous. She knew it was customary for therapists to work in this way, but that only showed how out of touch the profession was with people's lives.

I sensed she was still holding back, and I invited her to continue.

"I haven't formulated my thoughts, and I don't want to keep blurting stuff out."

"Sometimes the truth likes to be blurted out."

"I don't know! But I can't help thinking how hard most people in this world work for one hundred ten dollars. That includes the people in my family; they work hard for that money! Can you really appreciate it, coming from your background? It just hurts somehow that even with someone like you, there comes a limit between black and white, a limit of understanding."

Few things are as unnerving as confronting one's own racism, or being described as insensitive to race. I felt embarrassed and sad, but also encouraged by her willingness to speak her mind. I wondered if she had felt this limit at other times in our work.

"Last year, a college friend of mine told me her therapist was black, and it made me curious, you know, about the difference that might make. But, no, I have never felt until now that there was this limit between us. Like, 'You just don't get me.'"

We talked a bit about her fantasy of what it might be like having a black therapist, and exactly what it was about her that I wasn't "getting." We had reached the end of the hour, and I mentioned that we didn't have to wrap this up in one session. We could (and we did) return to the question of race and its meaning in our relationship.

Pearl was right about limits. No white person, regardless of sympathies, based or not on some shared experience of bigotry or poverty, can know from the inside the experience of any person of color. Race matters, and we err profoundly in not acknowledging the gap. And no therapist can understand any patient fully, even when their race and class backgrounds are similar. That we are fairly guaranteed to misunderstand each other is a useful if humbling truth. Psychoanalytic therapy is devoted to marking our longing for clairvoyant love, and our difficulty in recognizing all others as other.

As for the rules about time and money, it was clear to me that Pearl never would have allowed herself that candor had I not decided finally to apply my policy. To proceed along unspoken lines such as "How can I charge this poor black woman?" was, I realized, a countertransference problem, a simple rescue fantasy. Perhaps if I could grant her the privilege of not paying, her life would have less privation, her playing field would feel a bit more level. . . .

As we have seen in the other cases, a "resistance" to making the unconscious conscious belongs to the therapist as well as to the patient. For both, there is a yes and a no, always. I saw my not charging Pearl as a bit of resistance to doing the work. That is, sensing that Pearl was expressing anger or resentment through her no-shows, I nonetheless chose to let them pass, rather than invite her criticism. It was an act of self-protection. Realizing this made me flash on the story she had told early on about the racist white clerk who lined their hats with tissue paper to "protect" the heads of white customers. All therapists at some moment with every patient construct a kind of protective lining to shield themselves from what is going on inside the patient's head. One wants to know and yet one also does not want to know. . . . Unique to psychoanalytic training

is the emphasis on disciplining oneself to face rather than disavow one's own resistances.

What if Pearl had had a black therapist? Race would still
have mattered, but differently, as the experiences of therapists
of color have shown. The psychoanalyst Kimberlyn Leary, for
example, writes of her experience with African American patients who worry if she is "black enough" (or, perhaps, "too
black"). Race operates in therapy also when both patient and
therapist are Caucasian. I had a white patient years back who
periodically entered my office slinging racist criticisms of our
black receptionist. In minutes the patient and I would be in a
heated and thoroughly unproductive debate about racial
stereotyping. One day I saw a pattern: She always made these
comments when she was actually angry at me—for being late,
changing her appointment time, or simply pushing her too
hard to talk. This woman found it nearly impossible to get mad
at someone she liked. It was much nicer to think of joining
with me against someone who seemed to her an easy target.
My interpretation about her use of race marked a turning point
in our therapy.

·   ·   ·

In the week that followed our discussion about the fee, Pearl
phoned to apologize about spouting off. She seemed surprised
to learn that I was not irritated with her, and that I was no less
pleased to see her the following week. This helped her to understand that getting angry with close friends, with Joshua, and
maybe even with her mother might be possible. Porcupine-style
withdrawal was not the only way of negotiating distances in
love.

Pearl was enjoying her new relationship, her friends, her teaching. She was not at all sure, however, that she would remain at the university. On some days, she felt an ethical imperative to stay. There were now three graduate students who had chosen the department because they wanted to work with her, and their needs haunted her days. At other times, she felt she had to leave because she could never be happy at an institution of that kind. For the first time, her happiness was allowed to matter.

Pearl arranged to take an unpaid leave of absence to finish her book and discreetly look for other jobs. She would spend most of that time working in Africa with Joshua, and meeting his family. They were committed to each other, although the relationship had its sticking points, notably the question of children. Joshua wanted eight. "Now it's true that that's seven or eight more than I want, but he's not implacable. I'll bargain him down before long, you'll see."

Pearl knew we had not solved all her life's problems and that the question of kids was serious. She had never really considered being a mother until she met Joshua, she said. She felt sure he would be an involved parent, and that she wouldn't be sacrificing everything if they had a family.

Before she left the country, we cut our sessions back to every other week and then every third. Pearl cried like a little girl the day we said good-bye. She gave me a packet of her writings inscribed in a tender way. I heard nothing from her for nearly a year. Then one spring morning Pearl called saying she was back in the U.S. and wanted to say hello. I was delighted to greet her in my office.

She had loved her time in Africa, and pulled out photos of herself dressed in gowns of kinte cloth and standing next to a handsome man with very black skin. She had finished her book and written some poetry as well.

And what had she decided to do about her career?

She had accepted a job at a college in Georgia—a place less prestigious than the one she had left, but one that promised to be more rewarding. They valued teaching.

The matter of children—How many? Adopted or biological? And when?—remained unsettled. And then there was the question of her mother. Mrs. Quincey wanted to move closer to the couple, and although Joshua liked the idea, Pearl wasn't so sure.

I looked at Pearl. She was so different that day from the woman who had entered my office more than four years ago. Then she had been wracked with an inflamed sciatic nerve, lonely, insomniac, ruminating over obsolete words for grief— indeed, living with an obsolete self-description. Now she appeared vital, relaxed, hopeful.

I asked if she would allow me to include her in a book I hoped to write about psychotherapy. She gave an emphatic "yes!" as though a weight had been lifted.

"Our work has made so much possible: my book, finding Joshua, surviving my tribulations. I would love to give something back to you."

And so she did.

5   THE SIN EATER

EIGHT DOLLARS and ten cents an hour. That's what we, a top-notch team of psychologists and social workers, were earning in the early 1980s at our world-famous children's hospital and community mental health center.

I had been simmering quietly over this for some time, never reaching full boil until our director called a special meeting. Dr. Claude Bradley wished to announce that our caseloads would be increased by 20 percent, effective immediately. Were there any questions?

I raised my hand.

"We're working twelve-hour days as it is, Claude. Some of us are still in analysis and many have spouses and kids. I calculated my hourly wage last night, and here is my comment: I can't believe the amount of work I'm doing now for eight dollars an hour, and I'm not dying to do more."

No one moved.

"When did *you* get a raise?" came a voice behind me.

That would be Jeff, the class clown.

Claude was sympathetic. He was a decent, overworked guy who could have been making a mint in a different setting. He reminded us, as if we didn't know it, that we had chosen to work there because we valued community service over salary. Innovative programs and clinical seminars were the only other reason people had ever worked where we did, and that was not going to change. Mental health was no longer a national priority; his budget had been cut, and a chill wind blew. . . .

We had heard doomsday rumors for a year, but no one but Claude believed them. Looking back, I see that even he could not have imagined what lay ahead: a total dismantling of public mental health services. There would be huge layoffs of staff and, for the patients, a new world of crisis management usurping the old ethic of prevention and care. Claude was a good man, an able clinician, and someone who generally looked out for us. He had, I thought, a special affection for me.

"To all of you, I want to say I'm sorry about this. And to Luepnitz I would like to add: Cut the bellyaching."

There was more.

In recognition of our low salaries, the clinic would allow us to see private patients and keep 70 percent of whatever fee we wished to charge. If there weren't enough affluent clients to go around, we could work evenings and weekends at the satellite clinic in a wealthy suburb, fifteen miles away. This option was obviously more appealing to people with automobiles.

For the administration, private practice was a magic bullet. For this group of clinicians, it was a sell-out. Many of us had been active in radical politics in college, and all were influenced by the people-before-profits ethos of the sixties. Odd as it now may appear, many of us found the idea of seeking monied patients unseemly.

"I came here to work with people from my neighborhood, Claude," I said pointedly. "Rich folks will always be able to find the help they need."

"This is the eighties, Deborah," he countered. "Are women allowed to have good business sense yet?"

That was all Dr. Bradley chose to say.

I took off for the cafeteria, followed by Fran, my supervisor of many years. Times were changing, she said. One could treat rich and poor patients alike, no? One could be a force for social change without wearing overalls and living like a hobbit, right? It wasn't necessary to charge astronomical fees like some of the downtown shrinks, she added. Charging even half the going rate would make a huge difference. Just practice saying it, she urged in only half-jest. "My fee is fifty dollars."

I was shocked to hear her pick up where the boss left off. This was unpretentious Fran from Brooklyn, the anti-Yuppie, she of the oversized blue sweater we occasionally threatened to burn. And my favorite line, "Rich folks will always be able to find the help they need. . . . " Where did she think I got that in the first place?

Fran and I agreed to disagree.

Later that spring, my west Philadelphia apartment building was sold. The new landlord painted the lobby and doubled the rent. I began to think differently about things, including what my old mentor had said. Surely one hour of private service per week couldn't hurt. I practiced: "Good evening. I am Dr. Luepnitz, and my fee is fifty dollars."

I sashayed into the intake office one afternoon to request a 9:00 P.M. private patient. A teenager buying condoms would have sounded more confident.

"Could I please have . . . let's see . . . someone *professional*, or who . . . can afford, you know. . . . "

Two weeks later, intake assigned me one "Ms. Green," age twenty-five. Ms. Green had left a job she liked in Chicago to follow her fiancé to Philadelphia, but he had broken their engagement. She was depressed and looking for long-term treatment. Marion, the intake worker, had written at the bottom of the form: "Professional who can afford, *you know.* . . . "

The big night arrived. I wore my first-interview pantsuit and wrapped a pretty scarf around my neck. It had been hot and dry in Philadelphia for weeks, but on that July evening, the skies opened, catching everyone by surprise. By nine o'clock, people were entering the building soaked.

"There is a very drenched patient here to see you," said the temp who was answering phones.

I went out to greet Ms. Green, a tiny woman with a broken umbrella. She was only four feet eleven inches tall, and her jeans and sweatshirt made her look younger than her age. Her blonde shoulder-length hair was plastered behind slightly prominent ears. The wind had played rummy with her parcels, so that she looked more like a homeless person than like a center-city professional.

She was well-spoken and engaging, pausing occasionally to ask if she were going too fast, or to offer me a cigarette. Her mouth quivered as she began to speak of Enrique, the man who had left her. So fresh was the betrayal that she had not had time to drain the tenderness from her voice when she said his name. She bowed her head as Catholics do at the name of Jesus. *Enrique.*

Then she mentioned her daughter, Inez, whom I did not remember from the intake sheet.

I allowed her to continue, even as I realized that, not only was she not a high-salaried professional, she was one of the most down-and-out patients I had ever seen. She was, for example, homeless.

"I have an address, but not my own home; let's put it that way."

On the form, she had written the street number, but not the name of the shelter where she was living. She assured me that she had been there only two weeks, and did not intend to stay much longer. Ms. Green had lived in nice apartments in her life. She had been homeless only once before, and that was in Chicago as a young woman, long before her daughter was born. (For reasons I never fully understood, she did not count the year she lived at the post office.)

"Margie at the shelter gave me your name."

Margie was a Penn student volunteering at the shelter. Apparently, she had heard me give a talk on the importance of providing long-term insight-oriented psychotherapy to everyone who needed it, including low-income people. My argument was that only the sheerest prejudice made therapists believe that the poor had no unconscious conflicts, or that money made human beings more reflective. Margie had taken a liking to Ms. Green, and wrote down the clinic's phone number, suggesting she ask for "Deborah or Fran."

"Margie said this place was terrific. She said you stick with people and help them get their lives together. She said you let whole families live here to work on their problems."

"Ms. Green, did our office mention the fee?"

"Yes. She said that people who can't pay or have medical assistance are put on a waiting list in a different department. But I told her 'no problem' because I can pay."

"You *can?*"

"I worked last week. Thank you for not looking shocked. You know that a lot of homeless people have full-time jobs, don't you?"

Actually, I didn't. I learned only later that 20 percent work full time—that employment is no guarantee against homelessness.

"I got paid tonight. What will this cost all together?"

My tutoring kicked in, on cue. Sounding more like I had been abducted by aliens than not, I said, "My fee is fifty dollars."

"That's perfect!" she said. "They told me to count on a year or so of treatment, right? That's about a dollar a week. So here you go."

She plastered a damp dollar bill on the round table between us, and ironed it a few times with one tiny hand.

Surely this was happening to someone else.

"What do your patients call you?"

I wanted to say, "Fran."

"If I call you Dr. *Loo*-pen-itz, it takes too long and I won't call you anything. Using your first name would be too much like friends. What if I call you 'Dr. L'? Would that work? And please don't call me 'Ms. Green.' Use my first name."

I was struck with how seriously she was taking our relationship. Her first name was a name that connotes sadness. I will call her "Emily."

Formalities concluded, Emily asked if she might plunge in and talk about what had recently happened to her.

What had happened was that her heart and soul were cleaved in two by the only man who ever loved her. She had previous boyfriends in her life, but each one had mistreated her. One had beaten her with a hammer. Another stole her camera—the last thing she owned that belonged to her mother.

Enrique Marron, in contrast, was wonderful. Other men had called her "half-pint" and "Thumbelina." Enrique called her his "china doll." He taught her how to fix cars. He also helped her get the best job she had ever had, working for the post office. Enrique had already discovered that since the main branch was open twenty-four hours a day and was equipped with lockers and showers, living at work was a practical solution to tough times. Before they were lovers, they were friends and room-mates of sorts at the P.O.

Enrique, unfortunately, had a habit. Actually two habits: liquor and cocaine. Emily was clean, and had enough money to rent a small place for them. She was thrilled to have his child, and they named her Inez on his suggestion. It's true that he would go away for long stretches on business, but when he returned to Chicago, he was always happy to see them.

Emily had lost every bit of family she had by the age of sixteen. She had been hungry, battered, and neglected. Enrique was the proof that all could still be well. He said they would be married when he returned. Just around the corner, she saw a happy family, a special bliss.

Between choking sobs, she told me the final chapter. Enrique had been away too long. He phoned one night and said there was trouble; he would send for her when it got straightened out. She was afraid for him, and spent half the money she had on earth buying a bus ticket to Philadelphia. She was greeted at the door by his wife, the mother of his four other children. This woman began screaming in Spanish before bolting away from Emily and returning with an obviously loaded revolver. Enrique wrested the gun from her and pushed Emily out at the same time. He said he was the father only of the four children she had just seen. They were being evicted, and he was taking them back to the Dominican Republic.

Emily had hyperventilated for an hour. If not for Inez, shaking in her arms, she would have run in front of the nearest truck. She had no interest in the fresh hell that would be her life henceforward. Her lover was gone; her child had no father. They would never see him again.

Mother and daughter spent the night in the bus station at Eleventh and Filbert, where they ate crackers out of the vending machine and slept curled together on a plastic chair. When Emily awakened, her wallet was gone.

"Ripped off! In the city of brotherly fucking love!" It was an abject story, and I realized I was hearing just the outlines. She wanted me to know that Inez had been a happy child, but was miserable and withdrawn living in the shelter. This dirty, noisy place was enough to scare any child, she said. All night long they heard women going in and out of the bathroom, talking and arguing. There was one woman who would scream about Home Depot reading her thoughts.

"I need help being a good mom; I need help with a lot of things, but the first is falling out of love with Enrique. My father left when I was seven; my mom was a saint, but she died when I was ten, and my grandmother died sleeping next to me. Still, nothing hurt like this hurts. I hate to tell you this. I'm ashamed. But I was pushing that woman's arm—his wife's arm—because I wanted the gun to go off. I wanted her to kill me. Do you think I'm evil to think for a second of abandoning my kid? I'm not that bad. I need to hear from you. I need to know what you think of me."

I told her what I was thinking: that she had survived more pain in a few decades than many people did in a lifetime. I couldn't help commenting on her strength.

"People have called me a lot of things in my life, but not 'strong.' Thank you for. . . . Look. I would like to promise you something, OK? Help *me*, and I will take care of *her*," she said, pointing to the empty chair beside her. "Will you do that?"

Almost without thinking, I said I would. Of course.

I suggested Emily bring Inez to our next meeting, and she seemed relieved. Then she added, "Write down the time of the appointment, please. We'll be here unless I decide I can't stand this hick town another day. If you don't see me, you'll know we've headed out."

She stood up.

As I watched her fold her appointment card in two and use it as an ashtray, I wondered if I would ever see her again. It would have made life easier if she had hopped a bus back to

Chicago. On the other hand, I already felt interested in her, worried about her little one, tied somehow to them both.

And so it came about that I agreed to do my best for her, for Emily. The name came to me that very night, and I know why. Emily is the name of the girl left on a woman's doorstep in a novel I had just read, Doris Lessing's *Memoirs of a Survivor*. The story is set in a vague postnuclear winter, in which daily existence consists of hunting down provisions and uncontaminated water. Gangs of adolescent boys roam the streets, preying on survivors. An unidentified man with a female child comes to the door of the narrator and says, before vanishing, "She is yours. You must take care of her."

I don't remember leaving the clinic that night and walking to the Chinese restaurant down the street. Nor do I remember ordering a large plate of something and eating every bit. I know that these things took place, because I recall seeing an empty dish and feeling too stuffed to open my fortune cookie. I was lost in thought about the failure of my first foray into private enterprise.

Emily was by no means the sickest or most helpless patient I had ever seen. On the inpatient service, I regularly dealt with children who had been beaten, burned, left on agency steps, or otherwise savaged by parents who had experienced the same or worse as children. The reason I felt dazed was that I had had a different kind of patient in mind. How to account for this reversal of fortune? Doris Lessing's protagonist takes in young Emily because she has no choice. I had a choice. I could have explained the confusion and escorted her to the other side of the building and never seen her again. Obviously, I was not ready to do it, to become a woman of business, a lady of the eighties. I would do that, or something like it, in time. At the moment, my loyalties lay elsewhere. I considered the possibility that I had chosen Emily almost as deliberately as she had chosen me, to remind me of who I was. This thought was helpful, but it did not—could not—diminish my disappointment, exhaustion, or my very real fear of burnout.

Emily did show up for her next appointment. And the next. We had as few as one weekly contact, and as many as nine, for the following fourteen years.

．　　．　　．

Emily and four-year-old Inez came on time for our next session. Because the little girl was tall for her age, and Emily so short, they gave the impression of being the same size. Emily wore black leggings and a baggy black top that nonetheless revealed a bosom much larger than the rest of her. Her eyes were the color of blue topaz, almost gaudy next to her skim-milk complexion.

Inez was the photographic negative of her mother. She had dark skin and huge black eyes that seemed by turns startled and vacant. She wore Tommy Hilfiger sweats and little Reebok running shoes. A rumpled white bow tied up her tired pony-tail. She sucked her thumb, rubbed her belly, and stared ahead as her mother spoke. Whenever Emily cried, Inez cried. Inez had a bad cold and possibly conjunctivitis as well. Emily wanted desperately for her to see a doctor, but she could not apply for medical assistance without identification, and could not send for her birth certificate without a permanent address.

My first intervention turned out to be as helpful as anything I would do in the first two years. I decided to continue to see Emily alone, so that she would not have to share me with Inez. I referred them as mother-and-daughter to a group run by a senior therapist and her two residents. For a two-hour period of time, mothers and their young children came together to do activities and talk. The premise of the group was that moms in trouble lose the ability to simply play with and enjoy their children. Each group also included time for the mothers to talk alone with each other, while the residents took the children to an adjacent room for their time together. Mothers saw that they were not alone in their struggles. They helped each other navigate the social service system, and many made friends for life.

In the meantime, Emily made it clear that she intended to take her individual therapy seriously. Sometimes too seriously. I don't mind being called at home when a patient is in crisis. Emily was in constant crisis.

> *Monday:* I have to at least try to see Enrique one more time. Should I take Inez with me?
>
> *Tuesday:* Someone traded me two Libriums for a cigarette. The first one relaxed me, but now I'm sick.
>
> *Wednesday:* If you thought Inez would be better off in foster care, would you tell me?
>
> *Thursday:* I cannot take the exhaustion of walking around with her all day. I just want to die.

During this first month of treatment, I realized that in order to work with Emily, I would have to take good care of myself. I decided to line up an extra hour of supervision per week. I phoned Grace Strauss, a woman outside our department with whom I had worked as a student a few years earlier. Emily signed a release allowing me to discuss our work with my former teacher.

Grace was a woman of fifty, a salty, take-no-prisoners variation on the earth-mother archetype. She had just a handful of platinum hair framing the peaches-and-cream complexion of a thirty-year-old. She was six feet tall and carried her extra forty pounds as well as someone can. She dressed horribly. Everything had fringe or bows or pom-poms. She was canny, generous, and brilliantly funny. People who had not been helped by other therapists found help from Grace.

Grace listened to me describe my accidental patient and laughed her good, horsy laugh.

"Let's see: This Emily is homeless at the moment. She was orphaned by age twelve, has a four-year-old daughter in distress, and was recently dumped by the man she loves. She was robbed of her cash and identification, has no relatives on earth, no friends in town, a therapist who hasn't had a real vacation since high school, and a supervisor recovering from cancer. This is a train wreck, Deborah."

Even from her hospital bed, Grace had done therapy and supervision. It was more than obvious that she would outlive us all.

"Say yes, Grace."

She said yes. Her supervision fee was fifty dollars. She would charge me twenty-five.

"That would be an hourly, not an annual fee, Deb."

"Very *not* funny, Grace."

She listened a bit more and said, "With patients like this, I think in terms of decades, not years."

Remarkably, this appalling news brought relief. Grace had the experience of going the distance with a lot of people whose lives were shattered early on. If I were willing to put in the time, we could all more than survive this experience.

·   ·   ·

Emily was often overwhelming in her demands, no less than in her needs. But she was also irresistible. One evening, she stopped a story midway to say:

"I think therapy is a great thing, if I understand the rules right. I mean, I get to keep talking about myself, and I can count on you to listen, right?

"That's right."

"And even if you've had a tough day, and I have nothing fascinating to say, you listen anyway."

"Of course."

"You don't talk about your own problems, you still pay attention to me."

"Ri . . . ight."

"I like it."

"Yes?"

"It's like being a *guy* on a *date!*"

Who wouldn't want to listen to Emily?

Enrique had finally left the country, but she was still thinking about him, night and day. She imagined taking a plane to the D.R. and pleading with him to acknowledge his daughter. Occasionally, she thought about throwing acid in his wife's face.

Before Enrique, before her years of loss and bad luck, she herself had been a happy child, she said. Her parents, would-be artists, were eighteen years old when they decided to have her. Immature, they were rebelling against their parents, especially his father, who was a marine. They lived in a fifth-floor walk-up and took turns waiting tables, doing their art, buying drugs, and caring for Emily. They smoked a lot of pot, and her father turned to methamphetamines in his twenties, and then to heroin. Her mother was lively and affectionate. Emily remembered the two of them playing dolls together for hours. She

watched her mother paint, and was even given her own tiny
canvases.

The problems started when she was five. Her mother would
get depressed and not leave her bed for days. Emily remembered crying in class in first grade, worrying about her mother
at home. There were scenes of the parents hitting each other.
And then her father moved out when she was seven. Her
mother, who had suffered for two years from a severe case of
mononucleosis, went to the hospital for several days of tests.
Emily was shipped off to her paternal grandmother's for a
week. She never saw her mother again.

"How exactly did she die?"

"Heart failure. She wasn't a junkie like my dad, but she had
done a ton of drugs by then, and she was in terrible shape."

Emily's grandmother hoped that the mother's death would
bring her son back to raise Emily. It did not. He was killed in a
motorcycle accident when Emily was twelve.

Fortunately, her grandmother was willing to keep her, and
fortunately, they got along well enough.

"You remind me of Gram," said Emily. "She was dark like
you, and she loved a good laugh. She was Italian; I bet you are,
too. Anyhow, she was calm and stable, different from my mom.
I was no trouble until I was fourteen. Then she sent me to a
shrink, who told her I had a borderline personality disorder."

At fourteen, Emily began writing on her arms and legs with
a razor blade. It was for attention, she said.

"I had gotten really fat that year, and I was generally miserable. Twenty pounds on me looks like forty on someone else. I
think I cut myself because I hated being a fat kid."

Emily was working well in therapy, and in the mothers'
group as well. Inez had seen a physician who volunteered at the
shelter; she was eating again and playing with the other kids.

Emily was phoning me at home less often, but still paged me once a day.

> *Monday:* I think I have body lice. You better check yourself, because I was sitting on your couch and hugging your pillow this morning.
>
> *Tuesday:* I had a nightmare that the woman next to us stabbed Inez. Can I tell you my dream?
>
> *Wednesday:* A woman from the mothers' group wants me to move in with her. Is this a good idea?

In the group, Emily had met Nesta, an Iranian woman with a daughter Inez's age. They had sought shelter from her abusive husband, a physician, and would be out as soon as a lawyer could help reclaim her bank account. She could afford to rent an apartment, but was afraid to live alone. Nesta liked Emily and said in group that Emily had "a beautiful soul." The mothers in the group loved the idea of their working things out together. If Nesta could earn good money at her teaching job, Emily could stay home with the girls, solving the childcare problem.

Emily had reservations about Nesta's religious convictions. She didn't like her views on alcohol, drugs, or homosexuality, either. However, Emily also realized that getting an apartment together would be the best thing for both of them and their daughters. Within days they had found a place.

I imagined that being in a safer environment would cut down on her calls to me. It did not. In fact, on two occasions she showed up, unannounced, in crisis. Both surprise visits happened to be in the evening, as I was leaving the clinic for a date. I felt I had no choice but to spend a little time with her. She was impulsive and at risk of hurting either herself or Inez.

She was not yet able to say, "I'm afraid you will abandon me as everyone else has, and as I fear I deserve." Instead she enacted her desperation, pushing me to the point that I dearly wanted to abandon her. Not a day went by when I didn't feel trapped by Emily.

Friday: Inez won't eat anything except M&Ms. Should I let this go, or force her to eat? I really need some help with this.

Saturday: You didn't call me back last night, and I'm a little worried. Maybe you went away for the weekend. Just call when you get back, OK?

Saturday: I'm starting to get more worried, because I don't think you would have left town without someone covering for you. If you get this, please call me, OK?

Saturday: Um, this is getting pretty damned frustrating, because your line was just busy. Look, if you're fed up and you don't want to see me any more, just tell me, and I'll fuck off.

Grace had a recommendation.

"I hate to say it, Deborah, because I know you're swamped, but Emily needs more than one session per week. She's asking you in the only way she knows how. This is not a person to whom you can say, 'I'm still here, I haven't forgotten you.' You need to show it. She'd be an idiot to trust you now, and Emily ain't dumb. What are you thinking?"

"That I want to run away from home."

"I've been there. . . . "

"This is, in part, how Emily feels every day. She does this unconsciously so I will get a real clue about how she goes through life," I said.

"You are terrific to take her on, Deborah. Neither you nor I like diagnostic labels much, but you can see why somebody called her 'borderline' at fourteen. You know the joke, right? 'How do you treat a borderline? Refer 'em!'"

Of all the disliked diagnostic labels, the term "borderline personality" particularly rankles. "Borderline" has a slippery, euphemistic feel to it. Many young women who carry that diagnosis have said they would rather be called "a just plain nutcase" or "a loony-tune." Emily was later to tell me herself that she disliked the label intensely, and asked me to explain it.

Vats of ink have been spilled on the subject of this diagnosis. Does it refer to a real condition? If so, is it treatable? What can be said about the etiology and prognosis?

"Borderline" is a term clinicians use to describe people who, psychologically, are somewhere between normal/neurotic and psychotic. Neurotics—that is, most of us—have our conflicts and symptoms, but we manage to function in work and love, for better and for worse, most of the time. Psychotics typically don't function at all in work or love. To be psychotic is largely to relate only to parts of the self—or to the world as an extension of oneself.

People labeled "borderline" function in the world, but their relationship to it and to others is severely impaired. They tend to be self-destructive and impulsive. Emily's history of self-mutilation, and her decision months back to spend her last dollar on a one-way ticket to see a man who was doing his best to elude her, would be considered typically "borderline" behaviors. The cause of this condition is considered to be severe damage in the early parent-child relationship. The key word associated with "neurotic" is "conflict"; with "borderline," it is "deficit." That is, while neurotics face difficulties in reconciling the demands of self with those of others, the "borderline" is in trouble at the very level of having or being a self. It goes without saying that people who carry this diagnosis have exceptional problems in adult relationships. That's why some experts believe that psychotherapy works for neurotics only. The "borderline," it is said, will be unable to trust the therapist and thus will hire and fire one helper after another. These patients won't be able to accept the "new deal" of constancy and care offered by the therapist, because they are always responding to the internal rejecting parents.

The following was true: Emily was impulsive and had been deprived of the conditions conducive to forming a sturdy sense of self. Her ability to form a therapeutic alliance remained to be seen. She had been rejected and abandoned, yes, but she had also had certain good-enough experiences with her mother and especially with her paternal grandmother. Could we build on these? Would she be able to stay the course if I were willing to manage whatever came up?

Most of the time I felt I could handle my feelings for Emily, but there were times I returned her attacks with sarcasm. On one of the many occasions Emily undertook to tell me how little I was doing for her, she floated the idea that her time could be better spent at a gym or diet center. Instead of interpreting her comment as a question about my commitment to her, I snapped: "When you're afraid you might hurt Inez, can you call Weight-Watchers?" I was ashamed.

Grace assured me she had said dumber things to patients, and recommended we reread Winnicott's classic paper "Hate in the Countertransference."

Winnicott is famous for defining the good-enough mother as "one capable of having a straightforward love-hate relationship with her infant." He conceived of what we might call the good-enough therapist in much the same way.

"Straightforward," clearly, is the operative term in the definition. It points to the importance of acknowledging feelings, not disclaiming or disavowing them. A mother who hates her infant or who hates being a mother but cannot bear to have this feeling may do any number of destructive things to conceal it, such as having more children to punish herself, discouraging all expression of emotion in those around her, or attempting suicide. The therapist who is unable to bear the combination of love and hate experienced for a particular patient remains vulnerable to an array of harmful behaviors, such as forgetting appointments or showing up late until the patient drops out, gratifying each and every demand to cover up the hate, or acting it out through angry comments. Winnicott maintained that mothers (and by analogy, therapists) who could accept their ambivalence as inevitable were far less likely to do harm than the deniers.

Grace conjectured that the therapist who had seen Emily at fourteen and lost her after three sessions could not manage his hatred for Emily's petulant, angry, possibly borderline teen-age self.

The holding environment that Grace (and indirectly, Winnicott) provided for me at this juncture allowed me to do the same for my patient. I felt a renewed warmth and curiosity about Emily, who jumped at the chance to schedule more appointments (at the ongoing rate of one dollar per session). This did eliminate unannounced visits, as well as decrease the number of crisis phone calls.

It was when we began seeing each other twice a week that Emily told me some of the most wrenching details of her story. As a girl, she had dreamed of attending college and becoming a teacher. Everything fell apart when her grandmother died. During tenth grade, Emily and Gram had made a habit of watching television together and often fell asleep in Gram's big bed. Emily woke up one Saturday morning to find her grandmother lying motionless and cold beside her. Unable to come to grips with what she must have known to be true, Emily lay back on her pillow to think. She actually fell back asleep and dreamed. She told me she dreamed she and Gram were skiing. The sun was glaring off the white snow and Gram said, "It's time to go in, Emily. We're too cold." She awakened a second time and lay close to her grandmother as long as she could.

Finally—it could have been ten minutes or two hours later—she leaned over and mechanically picked up the blue receiver and dialed 911.

"My sweet Gram died peacefully of a burst aneurysm. At least she didn't suffer. It was the perfect way to die—from her point of view. But I don't think you can imagine how shitty I felt. How scared. I was completely alone in the world; not one human being cared about me. I closed my eyes and tried to space out and not breathe, just in case it could happen that God would take me, too. That was the last time I prayed. There is no God, Dr. Luepnitz. If there was a God, I would have died then and there."

After the funeral, the parents of a school chum insisted on taking Emily in. She was welcomed as part of the family and was able to stay in school. But she was not part of the family; this she felt all too keenly. They made the right noises, but she could not test limits and know, as other kids do, that she would still be loved. She wasn't loved. She was a charity case.

"I started to steal stuff from them and stay out all night to prove they didn't really want me. They had no choice but to boot me."

This family spoke about Emily to the local minister, who then met with her and offered to take her in. He was a young man and told people to call him "Greg."

"He helped me with my homework, but he treated me more and more as a friend. He would say, 'Let's watch this educational program on television in our pajamas.'"

A ritual soon began of snuggling in front of the television, which led to his having her masturbate him.

"It was nice at first. He was handsome and smelled good. I thought it was amazing he could even stand me, given all the stuff I had done to the Jones family. Later, I just wanted to puke, but I couldn't say anything. My uncle had tried something with me, and I walked away. But with Greg . . . where would I go if I ran away?"

There was no one to tell. She was sure the police wouldn't have given her the time of day. She attempted several times to run away, so Reverend Greg had no choice but to call Social Services. Emily spent the last year of high school in foster homes.

Foster care is often the final step before homelessness. This is not because caring, competent foster parents don't exist; it's because many overburdened families take in children only because they need money. Too, young people know that when they are sent to foster care they have hit the bottom rung on the ladder, and they begin acting accordingly.

Emily was determined to finish high school, but she made life miserable for as many foster parents as she could before it was over. One evening, when a foster mom called her "lazy," Emily spent the entire night in an unlocked car, and got what she called her "first taste of freedom." The summer after graduation was particularly warm, and she slept under the stars in the park. No more foster mothers or pointy-headed social workers, no more creepy uncles or masturbating ministers. It was just Emily and her new street-friends bumming change by day and sharing provisions by night in Chicago's Hyde Park. She spoke of it with nostalgia.

"It's horrible to be homeless when you have a child. But that time back in Chicago on my own was good. You could spend your day in the library or in those bookstores that have little restaurants in them, where someone has always left behind half a French-bread sandwich or a piece of carrot cake. When they closed, and it got cold outside, you would go in and sleep in a shelter. When the crazy fucks and the boosters made you nuts, you went back outside and enjoyed your freedom until you started to freeze. It may sound crazy, but there is a rhythm of the streets. Do you get what I'm saying?"

Porcupine life. The real thing.

I had named her after a fictional character, left on a woman's doorstep. But now my patient reminded me of another Emily, the one who wrote: "The Soul selects Her own Society. . . . "

That Emily, the "Belle of Amherst," also wrote:

I am alive—because
I do not own a House—
Entitled to myself—precise—
And fitting no one else—

Emily Green's love of freedom helped me understand the next phase of her life with Nesta and their daughters. Their apartment, located in a safe neighborhood, was warm and well-equipped. Nesta was generous and companionable. Emily was not ungrateful.

"It's better," she said laconically. "I can't say it's nirvana."

Emily had had enough on her hands with one four-year-old in her charge. Two was more than twice the trouble. She called me more often now, and not only because she possessed her own phone.

Monday: Razi swallowed some powder that might be detergent or poison or anything, and the writing on the box is in Farsi. I can't get her mother on the phone. What should I do?

Tuesday: God forgive me. I smacked Inez today, and it felt so good I didn't want to stop. I locked myself in the bathroom so I wouldn't kill her. I need to talk to you.

Wednesday: Thank you for talking to me yesterday. I'm calm today. But you said something I didn't quite understand, and I can't remember what it is. Will you call me back today?

Wednesday: Never mind, don't call. I'll just handle this myself.

Thursday: Thank you so much for calling back yesterday. I'm sorry I screamed at you. I want to run away. Can't you give me some medication? I would like to talk to you today about this, if possible.

The truth is that there were no effective antidepressants on the market at that time. Her physician prescribed a low dose of Valium, which seemed to take the edge off her most brutal moods.

I wasn't hating her at this point, but I was extremely disillusioned. I had assumed that sharing an apartment would help her immensely. Instead, she was more depressed and irritable than before. Staying home all day was a stark contrast to street life. If she had once been too much on the move, she was now unbearably sedentary. With two screaming kids, it was impossible to read or talk on the phone. She found herself watching television and snacking.

The high point of her day was watching reruns of Rod Serling's *Night Gallery*. On one occasion she left a phone message about an episode called "The Sin Eater." She loved scary stuff, but this episode turned out to be really disgusting, and she wanted to know if I had seen it. This was one of the calls I elected not to return. If the theme were important, it would turn up in a session.

As often as Emily longed to run away, her greatest fear was losing her daughter. Grace and I had discussed this from the beginning. No one would have been shocked if she had ended up bruising one of the kids. Knowing her own potential, however, she was determined always to call me before she lost control. To have placed Inez in foster care preventively would have been the more violent alternative.

"You're disappointed that her situation has not brought more relief," Grace counseled. "It's obvious you've never been a housewife, Deb. It has driven many a woman nuts." Rates of depression, smoking, and obesity are higher for housewives than for women who do not stay home, Grace pointed out. I learned later that many homeless women who decide to get off the street gain twenty to twenty-five pounds during their first year in residence. Grace predicted things would improve when the girls started school. This turned out to be true.

It was during first grade that Inez began asking about her father. This caused Emily a lot of pain. She had stopped loving Enrique, but she had not yet stopped hating him. What should she tell her daughter?

I invited them to talk together in my office.

Inez: "Why can't we see or call him?"
Emily: "His wife doesn't want us to. You see, he hadn't really told her about us. They had been separated a long time, but then they decided to get back together."
Inez: "Is she a witch or something, Mom?"

Emily: "Is she a witch? I don't really know her, honey. I
think she went wild that night because she wanted Enrique to take care of her kids, and she was fighting for
them, just like I would fight for you. A mother is like a
lion for her cubs."

Inez: "Will we get a new daddy?"

Emily: "I don't know. The important thing is that we're a
family. I will always love you. That's forever. And
Nesta and Razi love you, too."

I spent a lot of time feeling exasperated with Emily. Occasionally, I was dazzled by her constancy and clarity. I watched
Emily and Inez cuddle and talk, and I imagined wonderful
things for this mother and daughter.

"Emily, I was just thinking what a lucky mom you are to
have Inez for a daughter. She's so smart. She asked those questions in a lovely way. Is it OK for her to ask you again some-
time if she needs to?"

"Inez can ask me anything anytime. And she knows I like to
talk, talk, talk."

"Inez, how are you feeling now?"

"Good."

"You're a lucky girl to have this mom."

"Do we get a gold star for being a great team or what?"

"You do! I'm proud to know you."

And the truth is, I was.

•   •   •

With both children in school, Emily went to work at a diner.
There she met Jimmy, a good-looking Vietnam veteran. She
was thrilled when he flirted with her, and chastened when he

said, "Better lay off the breakfast sausages. I don't like fat girls."

Emily had gained twelve pounds as a "housewife," and when she began to diet, she gained eight more. She had struggled with her weight in high school, nearly always feeling unattractive, out of proportion, even freakish. The day Jimmy spoke to her, she went into "high diet gear." She brought home meatloaf and potatoes for Nesta and the kids, and sat at the table eating an orange. Her mood waxed euphoric as she watched her body shrink. People started describing her as "delicate" and "waif-like." It was hard to get my mind around it: a former street person struggling to look like a waif to attract a man.

"It's a good rule of thumb, Deb, that no sector of the populace is any less crazy than the rest," said Grace.

I understood this, and appreciated Emily's resolve, even as I challenged her starvation diet.

"Women are crazy to do this, of course!" Emily agreed. "But I am grateful to Jimmy, because he is my motivation."

Jimmy did something for her that I would be unable to do: put her on a diet and crack the whip. This undoubtedly spoke to her longing to be disciplined by a caring father or mother. Some therapists try (and generally fail) to motivate an end to their patients' compulsive eating. Others, sensitive to the inordinate emphasis on thinness placed on women by the culture, back away from weight issues altogether. What psychotherapy can and ought to do is to keep in motion a conversation about symptomatic eating: its origins, its ups and downs, its overt and hidden satisfactions.

Emily agreed to talk about eating. She could identify the month and the year when she started dieting. It started with a group of girlfriends who would dare each other to starve all week and then binge together on weekends. Some had learned to make themselves vomit.

We worked on eating and body-image for several months, during which Emily reported a recurring nightmare. She was on her way somewhere—sometimes to school, sometimes to work or to my office—and she had to walk across "some disgusting thing." The substance could be dirt, feces, vomit, or some combination of the three, but it always assumed a square or rectangular shape, "like a mat." She had no associations at first. Mine ran along the lines of her former homelessness and the squalid places she had slept. The word "mat" occurred with increasing frequency until I finally asked her to say everything she could about "mat." The word meant nothing in particular, she said. It was just an ordinary object. Except that it was the name of her father's brother. This man—an alcoholic and ne'er-do-well who lived on and off with Emily's grandmother—had groped her a couple of times when she was in high school. Emily tossed it off, contrasting it with what the minister had done. After all, Matt had only grabbed her breasts a couple of times and stuck his hands down her pants. When she told him to cut it out, he did. Consciously, it was no big deal. He had neither threatened nor pursued her, and she did not lose a friend in the process.

Nonetheless, he was her uncle, and she a fatherless child.

"Can you tell me more about this man and your feelings about him?" I asked.

She remembered being curious about him at first, wondering if he could tell her things about her father, even hoping he might take an interest in her. But he seemed to regard her only as a nuisance, blocking his view of the television, and always eating.

"He called me the little blimp, and stuff like that. I think I was surprised he wanted to lay a hand on me."

That turned out to be the year her weight shot out of control. She ate whole loaves of sliced bread and cans of chocolate frosting. Her grandmother saw her bursting out of her clothes and had a fit. After Gram outlawed bingeing, Emily started cutting her arms and legs with a razor.

Emily had always believed she became depressed because she was fat. She had never seen it the other way around: that she got fat because she was depressed. And she had never linked this behavior to the "disgusting Matt." Consciously, Emily considered their interactions insignificant. Her dream life suggested otherwise. There was still a mess at her feet, blocking access to any number of desirable things: education, earning a living, getting help.

I asked if she had told her grandmother about Matt. Emily reminded me that the incident occurred in the 1960s, before people openly discussed such topics. There was no *Oprah*. There was no teaching kids about "good and bad touch."

"Again, this may sound weird to you, but I would not have known how to tell Gram, even if I wanted to. It was like there were no words to say it, believe it or not."

I believed it! I had spent seven years getting a Ph.D. in clinical psychology without hearing the phrase "sexual abuse" or the word "incest." Research has since shown that approximately one girl in six has unwanted sexual contact with an adult before she turns eighteen. This pervasive phenomenon—involving mostly female children and male perpetrators—was something society would not allow itself to know until the women's movement broke the code of silence. Within two years of media exposure, people were already complaining they were "sick of the topic," and had begun treating survivors as whiners on witch hunts.

Working on these issues in therapy did not cure Emily's eating disorder overnight. She was now accustomed to allowing her body to speak for her. She quickly regained the twenty "Jimmy pounds" she had lost. The extra weight made her feel more distant from him, less enamored and vulnerable. Another reason she gained the weight quickly is that Nesta had caught her purging and shamed her. Emily took extra pains to hide her behavior, but several months after her bulimia had started, the toilet backed up. Nesta said if she didn't stop, they might need to reconsider living together.

Emily was not one for ultimatums, and she swiftly informed Nesta that the street people she knew were kinder and wiser than 90 percent of the people who lived in houses. She would leave whenever Nesta wanted her to.

These reports made me nervous that a call would come from Emily very soon saying she had indeed decamped.

"That sexist bitch is not going to call me disgusting," said Emily. "I mean I like her a lot, and I love her kid almost like my own, but I will not be called disgusting. . . . "

The concept of transference does not apply only to the therapist-patient relationship. Emily was allowing Nesta to stand in for all the other people who had abandoned her—the foster parents, the minister, and Enrique, too. A lot of people had become fed up with Emily, and she was finally getting the chance to talk back. I pointed out that Nesta obviously cared deeply for Emily—that she felt the behavior was disgusting, not Emily herself. And she wouldn't have this reaction to Nesta if her words didn't ring true. Emily believed herself to be disgusting. And this, I said, was what we had to change. She was a good and lovable person, a wonderful mother, and someone to whom many people were drawn. I asked what she was thinking.

"When you say nice stuff to me, my first thought is to say, 'Cut it out. You're just jerking me around.'"

"And the second?"

"My second thought is: Don't stop. I love kindness. I remember the first day I came here and you called me 'a strong woman.' Christ, it made me want to live and make you proud of me."

Emily stopped vomiting to control her weight within months of our working on it. She mourned this part of her symptom as one does the loss of a particularly helpful friend. It had allowed her to soothe herself without gaining more weight than she could handle. Other thoughts nonetheless won the day: She did not want her daughter to become obsessed with food as she had been. And she was determined not to let her abusers win, by leaving so foul a trace.

.   .   .

There were stretches of time, months perhaps, when my relationship with Emily felt easy, collaborative. By the third or fourth year, I no longer thought of her as a child left on my doorstep. In the second year, she even raised the fee on her own to ten dollars an hour, and later to twenty.

A new countertransference challenge arose when her former landlord finally returned her security deposit of two hundred dollars. Emily had been complaining about being broke and having to forgo five-dollar arch supports for her aching feet, never mind Christmas gifts. When the check came, she proceeded to spend one hundred fifty dollars on a designer dress for Inez, and forty on Barbie clothes. That left ten dollars for utilities. She cursed a life that made it impossible to buy a pair of cheap arch supports. She would have to borrow money to buy Christmas gifts for Nesta and Razi.

Her improvidence infuriated me. I was offering therapy at next-to-nothing and buying my clothes in thrift stores. Not so, Barbie! Initially, I tried to convince Emily that she would be better off dealing with necessities first, but my unsolicited financial advice only made her feel she should keep quiet about such things. I soon realized that my role as therapist was not to teach thrift but to help her question the choices that kept her in a bind. In the early years, she had deflected such questions. As time went on, she was able to think critically about her use of money. She came to realize that a part of her desired financial turmoil.

"I am so used to it," she said disarmingly. "I wouldn't recognize myself if my bills were paid up. It wouldn't be *me*, if that makes any sense."

It did, of course, make plenty of sense. Living on the edge was so familiar that she could not possibly feel at home without some sense of external menace. It was easier to fight the electric company than the voices in her head that said, "You're lazy, you're a nuisance, and you don't deserve the good things you have."

This is the area where we focused years of our work. As for money, the only challenge I could actually leverage concerned her payment of me. She often fell months behind, but always eventually paid up.

•   •   •

Six years after Emily came to see me, I considered leaving Philadelphia for a new professional opportunity. The idea of moving to Boston both enticed and worried me, and I began drawing up lists of pros and cons. Emily always made the list.

"Of pros or cons?" Grace asked over cappuccino. Emily was doing better, and I was, too. Grace and I had met weekly for the first two years, but then tapered off. Although it had been months since our last meeting, I wanted to tell her about my Boston dilemma. Moving would mean not seeing my friends as often, but it would mean leaving my patients for good. Each one would face a difficult transition, but Emily might find it devastating to lose our relationship. I was the one person in her adult life who had cared for her continuously.

Grace took a strong stand. It would be difficult for Emily, yes, and she might have a crisis over it. But there were ways to prepare patients for such events. I could invite Emily to interview two or three potential successors and even try a few sessions with each of them. If I stayed behind for Emily, I would surely resent her.

"No one is indispensable, Deborah. Not even you or me!"

I did not move to Boston, but not because of Emily. The change I really needed was a good, long vacation. I made plans to visit a friend abroad, and began telling patients the dates of my holiday.

Emily was remarkably calm. She wanted to know where I was going, and I told her.

She was doing well. She was driving a school van by day and fixing cars on weekends. Inez was thriving. She was a lively ten-year-old, a fine student who was speaking very passable Spanish.

"Inez talks on the phone, earns money doing chores for the lady upstairs, and sits and counts her bucks at night. She's even loaned me money for groceries a couple times. Sometimes I look at her and have to think: 'Where did this child come from?'"

Emily said she was looking forward to three weeks without therapy. She needed time to get things done around the house. She wrote down the number of the person covering for me and borrowed a book from my shelf to have "something of you to hold on to." This was what we always did when I went away.

I was busy packing when Emily phoned the following morning. She was so sorry and ashamed. She had had a couple of beers and was feeling sorry for herself. She was so miserable about her life that she had downed a bottle of aspirin before calling me.

I sent Emily to the emergency room and finished packing. I hated her with great equanimity. She was my patient and I would always do the right thing for her. But she was still Emily: damaged, demanding, and maybe borderline Emily, who could not bear separation. I was not about to give anyone the power to ruin my holiday, however. This is why God made emergency rooms, Grace would have said.

We were able to have a session before my plane left. Emily said she had been calm about my going away until that morning. Nesta was away for the weekend and Inez was spending the day with her girlfriend. All she could think of was: What if the plane crashed? What if she never saw me again? What if I fell in love and decided to stay there? How would she live?

Emily had felt suicidal off and on during the six years I had known her (she was now thirty-one years old), but this was her first actual gesture since her teen years. Why now? It's true that I was going away for a week longer than I had in years past. Did that alone explain it? Or had she somehow intuited over the previous months that my leaving her for good had been a real possibility?

There was another, more cogent factor. I had overlooked an important anniversary in her life. Inez was ten years old—

precisely the age Emily was when her mother died. They said good-bye one day and never saw each other again. Planes don't crash every day, but in Emily's world, the people you count on do fall off the face of the earth. Her father had had an affair and left them behind, then her mother died, and then Gram.

It was in that emergency session that she spilled the truth about her mother's death. Her mother had overdosed on painkillers the week Emily was sent away, and she left a suicide note. Her grandmother could not bear to tell ten-year-old Emily the truth, saying instead that the death was caused by heart failure. The older woman considered this the whitest of lies: All deaths involve the stopping of the heart. When she told Emily the truth five years later, she recommended her own spin: People look down on suicides, she said. Don't tell anyone. It's no one's business, anyway.

Emily had revealed other painful and mortifying facts about her life. Why had she failed to tell me this one? It was, very obviously, the most wounding truth of all. It meant that she, Emily, was the kind of person that everyone, even a mother, could toss aside. Her mother's overdose followed not only years of depression but also continual threats of suicide.

"My mother used to say stuff like 'Some day I'll just put my head in the oven.' She would talk as if I wasn't in the room, but I was standing right there.'"

I wondered how she understood these words as a child. "I believed she could do something awful. I didn't know you could smother yourself with gas fumes. I thought she meant she would put her head in and cook it like meat. It pisses me off to think she would scare a kid like that! At that time I wasn't pissed off, I was just freaked. I would do anything, say anything, be good as gold, promise to take care of her forever, just so she wouldn't put her head in the oven."

I asked how her mother's mother died. Emily picked her lip for what seemed like minutes before saying she had died when her mom was just six. "Of 'heart failure.'"

Emily spliced this fact together with other things her grandmother had told her, and realized something she had never been able to acknowledge—that she came from not one but two generations of maternal suicide.

Now that she herself had a young child, she could not imagine how a mother could do such a thing. She had never threatened to hurt herself or run away in earshot of her daughter. She was embarrassed about her own overdose, but said it was just a stunt. There were only twelve pills in the bottle, and she had made herself vomit before she even phoned me. Nothing on earth, she realized, could make her do to her child what her mother had done to her.

Twelve is far below the minimum lethal dosage of aspirin, as we both knew very well. Nonetheless, I said, it should not be taken lightly. Perhaps she was trying, precisely, to understand how her mother could do such a thing. Emily had done this as a way of comprehending her own mother's incredible choice. That was the sense I made of her gesture, and I asked for her thoughts.

She said the pieces were beginning to fit together, and she wanted to write about it in her journal. While I was away, she would check in with the person covering for me at least twice a week. Could she perhaps have my phone number in Tunisia?

No, I said, that would not be possible.

It was time to stop. I reassured her I had every intention of coming back. She squeezed my hand and wished me a good trip.

I had a wonderful time away.

●　　●　　●

Emily was relieved to see me on my return. As promised, she had phoned the person covering for me, "just to touch base." In the ensuing six months, she did a lot of reflecting on why she had kept her mother's self-inflicted death a secret. It was a way of protecting her mother, she realized.

"My mom was a saint" was one of the first things she had said in therapy. Idealized parents often turn out to be abusive or seriously neglectful. Children (and adults) wanting desperately to believe that someone has loved them—that they are not the descendants of a bad race—produce a gilded picture of a parent and frame it for the world.

What does it do to a girl to grow up believing that any day, her mother might kill herself? Children blame themselves for all kinds of things, for parental quarrels, for illness, and, certainly, for divorce when it occurs. The suicide note was lost, and we could only guess what her last thoughts of Emily may have been. We do know that Emily spent her young life consoling her mother when upset, and acting brave when she lay in the dark crying. Perhaps as damaging as the mother's actual death was the strain of living every day—as another patient put it—"on red alert." Losing her mother through suicide meant that Emily could never believe anyone would stay attached to her. Furthermore, anyone who promised to do so incurred her wrath, precisely because they aroused hope.

Months later Emily was able to say how much she had despised me—the one person she had trusted not to abandon her—for going away when she needed me there.

Emily told me she had been "messed up" by her grandmother's tendency to let everybody off the hook. Gram had insisted that her mother was a tragic figure who died for love of her man. Likewise, said Emily, Gram had preferred to say that Emily's father was a sensitive guy whose own sadistic father had abandoned Gram and him. He fell into the wrong crowd, and the drugs did him in. He definitely would have come back to care for Emily had he lived.

Within weeks of my return, Emily began to express anger at the various protagonists in her early life. Yes, her parents and her uncle and Greg had had their own troubles, but they seemed in various ways to get off "scot-free." Her parents had never been held accountable for their behavior, nor had her uncle. And Reverend Greg? He was given a humanitarian award, married a beautiful woman with four daughters, and moved to Australia!

"Scot-free!" said Emily. She felt she was left behind to live a life of payment for their misdeeds.

"It's like in that TV show, *Night Gallery*," she said. "Do you remember me telling you about the sin eater?"

I did remember her mentioning it. Now I invited her to describe the episode.

This is the *Night Gallery* story as Emily remembered it: Each village in an unnamed country of a bygone era has its sin eater. When someone in the village dies, the corpse is laid out on a bier with bread, meat, and sweets on his chest that absorb his sins so his soul can go to heaven. The sin eater (always a poor person living on the fringes of the village) has the job of eating the food off the corpse, taking the sins on himself. In this episode, there is a famine in the land. A woman sends her son to act as sin eater at a funeral so he will not starve. In so doing, the child becomes an outcast; he cannot marry, and with no son of his own, he will have no one to take on his sins.

"The buck stopped with him. Is that sickening? Imagine eating food off a rotting corpse. Maybe you had to see the show."

"It really speaks to you, this story. You feel that you—"

"—ate all the crap they dished out: my mother's suicide, my father's drug addiction and womanizing, my pervert uncle's child-incest sins. No wonder I feel so goddamned bad. When I piss off Inez, she tells me about it! I was put through God-knows-what hell, and none of them has to hear about it. I have to have their misery and their voices in my head forever. *I'm* the sin eater."

She had found a metaphor for herself, deeply resonant. Emily felt poisoned by her past. She had taken in good things from her family, of course, but also their madness, pain, and just plain evil. She sometimes wanted to purge herself of "all things family." That, she said, was where the bulimia came in. When she vomited, she had a wonderful sensation of relief. The "bad" was out for a while. Sometimes she imagined "one great vomit" that would free her completely.

In later years, she was able to cobble together a more balanced image of her mother. She was neither saint nor evil incarnate. And while her own mother had died when she was only six, she had held out until Emily was ten—almost twice as long. And whereas she had been left alone with an alcoholic father, she made sure to leave Emily in the loving hands of Gram. Emily speculated that her mother's depression worsened after Emily started first grade, since that had been about the same time in her life that her own mother had died.

It was around this time that Emily spoke to me about a new drug she had heard of called Prozac. She had taken Tofranil as a teenager, but it proved useless. The drug gave her dry mouth and other side effects, but did nothing for her mood. Prozac was being touted as a miracle drug—an antidepressant that actually elevated mood and had only minor side effects.

I had read Peter Kramer's *Listening to Prozac*, and I was impressed. Emily struggled with depression each day. I saw no reason for her not to try it, so I referred her to a psychiatrist. Prozac and its cousins—the SSRIs—have reportedly helped millions of Americans, but Emily was not among them. A low dose had no effect, and a higher dose proved so stimulating she could not sleep. The psychiatrist added a sleeping medication, but it left her too groggy in the morning to drive a school van. Every six months or so, Emily would try a new drug, cooperating with the suggested titrations, but with equally poor results. Emily appeared to be among the group of Americans suffering from depression for whom no medication brings relief, a group estimated to number 3.6 million.

There was one side effect that Emily found immensely vexing, and she never let me forget it. While taking any antidepressant, she noticed a marked decrease in libido. I was surprised at the magnitude of her annoyance. Just because she didn't have a partner didn't mean she wanted to feel "neutered," she said.

"Who convinced America that having no sex drive was a 'minor' side effect? I mean, what is *wrong* with people?"

Sexuality became the focus of years seven to nine of her treatment. Emily spent a number of sessions complaining about Nesta's censorious comments about her gay friends.

"'Homosexuality is 'an a-BOM-mee-NAY-shun!'" Emily would say, mocking her roommate. I wondered if Emily were starting to question her own heterosexuality.

Emily had had crushes on female teachers and had done some adolescent experimentation with other girls. Her adult sexual encounters, however, had been only with men. She seemed to enjoy sex a lot, and could still speak fondly of her passionate nights with Enrique. Sometimes he had joked about a threesome, but she scoffed at the idea. Secretly, she said, it might have been nice.

"Does that make me a lesbian?"

Emily was still attracted to men, but she had been treated so badly by so many of them, she could barely stand the thought of trying again.

Emily loved women. She figured it would make life easier to sleep with the people she naturally enjoyed. She began spending more time with a lesbian friend from the mothers' group she'd attended years earlier. They made friends with others who frequented Giovanni's Room, Philadelphia's most established gay-and-lesbian bookstore. Was Emily going to come out as a lesbian?

In a word, yes.

Her unequivocal support of other people's gay relationships masked enormous ambivalence about her own desires, however. She was attracted to women, and nearly all of her sexual fantasies had been about women. Some of these fantasies were about watching two women make love; sometimes she herself was part of the scene.

There were only two obstacles to her trying a lesbian romance, she said.

"First of all, I can't understand the idea of being two things. If I'm attracted to men, how could I also be attracted to women?"

"What do you mean, how could you be? You are attracted to both."

"Yes, but how *could* I be?"

"Aren't some people bisexual?"

"Well, not me. I only want to be one thing."

"OK. Because being 'one thing' would be—"

"—better. *Easier.* It means you know who you are, you know what to tell people."

This was a complicated matter, certainly not made simpler by the political arguments she heard from various quarters. Nesta assured her that as long as she was attracted to men, she was "normal." Her lesbian friends said that so-called bisexuals were simply gays "afraid to come out."

"You said there were two problems with having a woman partner. What's the second?"

"The second problem is that it disgusts me. The idea of being with a real woman. I don't think I can do it."

Emily had come to realize that as much as images of women's bodies aroused her, she could not imagine having physical contact with an actual woman.

It came down to this: It's OK to love men, but I don't. I love women, but I don't desire them, except in fantasy. Moreover, I cannot bear ambiguity: I want to be *one thing*.

If there is any Freudian idea that has marked Western psychology indelibly, it is that human sexuality is never "one thing"—never a "natural" or unified masculinity or femininity. It was early on in Freud's career when he became influenced by Wilhelm Fliess's theory that everyone is born with a bisexual disposition. Freud's own terminology became more radical over time: He claimed that childhood sexuality was "polymorphously perverse." In the case of "Little Hans," for example, Freud pointed out that five-year-old Hans had erotic strivings toward not only his mother but also his father, and, in fact, fantasized getting pregnant by the father and giving birth anally. Voyeurism, exhibitionism, sadism, masochism—sexual urges in all their variants are present in what is sometimes called the "overinclusive" sexuality of children. Children start off wanting not "one thing" but, in a sense, everything and everyone. Civilization, by way of the family, encourages the expression of some urges and the repression or sublimation of others. The process through which the polymorphously sexual child becomes a "normal" heterosexual or homosexual adult, Freud called the Oedipus complex. Many lay people, and some therapists as well, remain unaware that Freud described two aspects of the complex: the positive and the negative. The words connote not good and bad but, rather, a thing and its inverse, like a photograph and its negative.

In the positive Oedipus complex, a child desires exclusive possession of the cross-sex parent and longs to displace the other parent. But each child also desires the same-sex parent and longs to displace the other. Freud changed his mind about certain things in the course of his career, but never this one. In his *Three Essays on the Theory of Sexuality*, he wrote:

> [A]ll human beings are capable of making a homosexual object-choice, and have in fact made one in their unconscious. . . . Thus from the point of view of psycho-analysis, the exclusive sexual interest felt by men for women is also a problem that needs elucidating and is not a self-evident fact.

Although Freud did not say so explicitly, we might think of heterosexuals as those for whom the positive Oedipus complex dominates and homosexuals as those for whom the negative Oedipus complex dominates.

In a 1935 letter to a mother concerned about her son's sexuality, Freud replied:

> Homosexuality is assuredly no advantage, but it is nothing to be ashamed of, no vice, no degradation; it cannot be classified as an illness. . . . Many highly respected individuals of ancient and modern times have been homosexuals, several of the greatest men among them (Plato, Michelangelo, Leonardo da Vinci, etc.). It is a great injustice to persecute homosexuality as a crime—and a cruelty, too.

Most unfortunately, however, Freud's successors elected to dismantle his Oedipal model and its ethic. The American Psychiatric Association classified homosexuality as a pathological condition until 1973.

Most, although not all, American analysts have changed with the times—becoming more open to "nontraditional" sexual relationships. Books on sexuality by psychoanalysts who are themselves gay or lesbian have done a great deal to de-pathologize homosexuality. Some practitioners, such as feminist Kim Chernin, go so far as to suggest that the ultimate aim of psychoanalytic treatment might be the restoration of the patient's "full bisexuality."

Emily realized that Nesta's criticism of homosexuality as an abomination hit a nerve. Emily herself worried that same-sex love was "unnatural" and once speculated that her attraction to women was a punishment for some crime (unknown) leveled by a vengeful God (in whom she didn't believe).

We worked through these matters painstakingly, separating clotted questions, fantasies, and beliefs. First there were the practical present-day concerns she had about her own safety, and that of Inez. If she were to start dating women, would they become victims of hate crimes? Would Inez be mocked at school? Would Inez turn against men? The simple articulation of these questions brought some relief, and talking to gay friends with kids helped even more. "Inez has such a strong mind of her own," Emily concluded. "She gets along fine with the boys and men in our life. As for safety—I guess we've made it through worse stuff than homophobia."

On the "middle shelf" (Emily's phrase) were memories of Gram and Gram's values.

"My grandmother and her friends shared a hairdresser for fifteen years. He knew how to fuss over them, Maurice did, but he was gay, and I mean, gay as a French parade. I could always get a laugh out of Gram by prancing around like Maurice. But in high school when I started hanging around this one teacher who looked butch—I don't even know if she was a lesbian—Gram went nuts. She started in with 'The Bible says "homos" are dirty and sick.'"

Emily's reminiscence ended in one short, sad statement: "If Gram were alive, I could not date women."

I wondered if the converse were true. Did not dating women keep Gram alive in some way? I raised the question with Emily.

"Yeah. It's like I keep her alive by thinking she's watching me and deciding what I can or can't do."

There was no telling what Gram would have thought of homosexuality if she were living now, Emily realized. We talked about the possibility of keeping her love alive, without living in fear of her judgments.

There was a "third shelf" to Emily's fear of loving women, and that one contained thoughts and feelings about her mother. There were times when her mother forgot to kiss her good-night, or did so perfunctorily because she was drunk or high. Emily would "pay her back" by refusing to kiss her on the nights she did want affection. After her death, the memory of having denied her mother kisses haunted Emily.

"It was the worst part about her dying. When I thought of how I used to send her away, hurting her feelings on purpose, I just wanted to puke. Nothing I have done in my life made me feel as guilty as sending her away."

Emily had told me many times that the idea of kissing another woman "disgusted" her. That is, it evoked the same physical sensation as rejecting her mother did. Loving another woman seemed impossible, perhaps, because its unconscious meaning was a permanent replacement—an absolute rejection of her mother.

As we worked through these feelings, Emily felt the taboo on her desire give way. She came in one day with a dream she couldn't possibly tell me. It was the most embarrassing thing imaginable. She had dreamed of making love with me.

"I don't wanna gross you out. I mean, I'm sure you're straight, and you've never wandered around like an idiot saying, 'I wonder what I am. I wonder what I am.'"

Grace had commented early on about the erotic side of Emily's transference to me. Feeling like "a guy on a date" with me revealed more than her saucy humor, although this did not need to be interpreted right away.

Emily was relieved that I could listen so matter-of-factly to her dream. I reassured her that sexual feelings for therapists, while never to be acted out, were acceptable, interesting, and useful to our work.

My comfort with her sexual feelings for me seemed to grant Emily permission to accept her desire for other women. She returned to her fantasies about me only near the end of our work together.

"I always thought you would be the perfect partner. Everyone wants someone like you who listens, who is generous, and pretty, and smart. But I was thinking the other day that—no offense—I feel that way because I don't really know you. If I did, I might think you were a pain in the ass like everybody else."

I couldn't have said it better.

More attention to her sexual feelings led her to describe a fear of being bitten during oral sex. Many of her erotic fantasies were absolutely ruined by this particular image. She had enjoyed oral sex with her male partners, and had no actual memory of being bitten or biting. Her lone association was another memory related to her mother. Her mother had tried to nurse Emily, but weaned her abruptly—so the family lore went—because she was a biter. The guilt Emily felt about rejecting her mother as a child—and even as an infant—was interfering with her adult sexual possibilities. The fear of being bitten was again the fear of reprisal for her own "attacks" on her mother's body.

After many months of work on these issues, and after reading many books on coming out, Emily had sex with a woman. We were eight years into our work when she began a serious relationship with Amy. Amy was six years younger, a college graduate who had grown up with liberal parents and who found Emily fascinating. She saw Emily as a street-wise woman, someone instinctively political. Amy convinced Emily to take some community college courses. Emily got Amy to loosen up and apologize less.

"We're good for each other, I think. But the main thing, I have to say, is the sex. It's the best. Enrique, you know, would say, 'Not tonight; I'm so tired.' Amy is always hot to trot. She is amazing. We were both late for work the other day. Ask me if I cared!"

Emily announced that while she might be "technically" bisexual, she was, as far as the world was concerned, henceforth and for all intents and purposes, a lesbian. And proud indeed.

Inez was eleven when Amy came on the scene, and, predictably, she threw some tantrums. By thirteen, Inez had made her point of view clear to her mother, and Emily quoted Inez to me:

"*God*, Mother, she's so *white*. Did you see her eating french fries with a fork? I think it's cool you're a lesbian, and Amy is a nice woman; she's just a *geek* is all I'm saying."

"Inez sounds OK, like a normal kid, doesn't she, Dr. L?"

"Totally," I said.

Things soon turned around between Inez and Amy; they actually became close after the three of them started sharing an apartment. One night Emily asked if they could have a family session: for herself, Amy, and Inez. They had been having loud arguments, and Emily was feeling left out, as Amy and Inez— the two intellectuals, the two neatniks, the two people who would never part with a dime—took sides against her in the business of everyday living.

Amy and Inez pled guilty, and the session was lighthearted. Emily told me the following week that she had mostly wanted me to meet her partner and to see Inez all grown up.

And then she cried, like someone leaving a friend at a train station, like someone saying good-bye for good. She said, "I can't bear sometimes to think of how thankful I am to you. I was looking at Amy, who has been so good to me, and looking at Inez, this healthy human being, and thinking: 'This did not have to be! In fact, I could be dead, I could have AIDS, my little girl could be dead. What if we had not found that shelter? What if Margie had been sick that day?' I know very well that I've worked hard, but you have, too. I will always be thankful to you, Dr. L, and I will think of you every day as long as I live."

Emily was not ready to stop therapy; she was not even suggesting it. But she apparently needed to punctuate our work in this way. It was a comma, not a full stop. Certain questions had been answered. Yes, she could raise a child who was competent and self-respecting. Yes, she could find an emotional home in the world.

Emily and Amy lived together for five years. What broke them up, predictably, was the question of more children. Emily felt she had used up every bit of her luck raising one child who had turned out OK. She was not about to tempt fate. Amy, for her part, could not imagine living life without children of her own. They remained close friends, even after Amy found another partner.

An interesting thing happened as Emily mourned this important relationship: She did not revert to bingeing in order to put space between Amy and her. This had been the quintessential porcupine symptom, in my view. Emily used her pounds as quills, deploying them to keep people at bay, retracting them to get close. Perhaps, by the age of thirty-six, she was tired of using her body in that way. She had developed better coping stratagems, including one that we associate with another kind of pointed quill: Emily had begun to write.

She wrote in a journal, she wrote and rewrote papers for her courses, and she even submitted a piece to a local magazine.

A copy of *Street News*—a New York City newspaper created and distributed by homeless people—fell into her hands. Emily was thrilled to read it. She showed me an Ann Landers–type column in the paper called "Ask Homey." The column offered answers to frequently asked questions about homelessness.

"I could do that! Why couldn't Philadelphia have a paper like that? There are thousands of people living on the street here."

No such paper materialized, but Emily continued to hone her skills.

She also continued to date, but didn't get deeply involved with anyone. She was absorbed with her studies, and adored her teachers. She was making a reasonable income as a car mechanic. Emily was a woman on the move. She decided that romance would come when it would—or not. She could imagine falling in love again, but she was not about to fall apart without it. A single life would not be a tragedy, she said. The only disaster in life would be to find yourself stuck with someone you didn't really love. At the moment, she had a full agenda and a daughter who still needed raising.

Emily was reading more each year, and had a habit of relating to her life every book she touched. No theme ever resonated more with her, however, than that of the sin eater. It pulled together her symptoms (bulimia and compulsive eating); her pain's history (the sins of the fathers and mothers); her experience of herself as performing a service (containing the distress of others); and her own personal aesthetic, for she loved the macabre. The image was both abject and noble, repulsive and essential, an identity "meant to be," yet one she could take upon herself to change.

Sin eating was more than that: it was a bit of original theory she used in order to understand a widespread social phenomenon. After she read about the epidemic of eating disorders in our country—a trend that was catching on in Europe and even India—she fulminated:

"Women eat because it's what we did in our families. We had all their shit stuffed down our throats. How many fat girls are sin eaters?"

It was a question worth asking.

There was another story going through my mind at this point, also a story about funeral rites: that of Antigone.

The daughter of Jocasta and Oedipus, Antigone breaks the civil law by performing a funeral rite for her fallen brother, a traitor. She is imprisoned by her uncle, the king, and hangs herself in jail. Scholars from Hegel and Kierkegaard to Freud and Lacan have commented on Antigone from points of view philosophical, psychological, ethical. The obvious is always overlooked: Antigone repeats her mother's act. Jocasta also dies by her own hand, and also by hanging.

Emily's mother, like Antigone, followed the path of her own mother in suicide. Emily's most brilliant gift to her child was rejecting the legacy of despair, thus—we can hope—breaking the cycle of tragedy.

One day during Emily's final year of therapy, a delayed Amtrak train caused me to miss our appointment. I had no way of contacting her, and I felt awful imagining her at my door, growing worried, getting angry, storming home. Surely, I thought, this will not trigger a crisis, although it might throw her off for a week or two.

As soon as the train pulled into the station, I phoned Emily and was shocked to find her warm and equable. Of course, she said, there was a chance something bad had happened to me. It was much more likely, however, that I had been delayed by an emergency with another patient and would call as soon as I was able.

I hung up the phone and needed to sit down for a few minutes. It is at times like this that therapists feel the earth move. It's not when the big revelations tumble out, or even the times when the patient effuses gratitude. The most satisfying moments are these seemingly mundane occasions that make one feel a person's molecules have been somehow rearranged for the better. I felt that all the time, patience, skill, compassion, and money I had put toward the healing of Emily had reached her, and not only reached her but settled into a kind of emotional bedrock. Whereas in the beginning she had to contact me every day just to confirm that I knew her, and whereas when I went away for three weeks she had not been able to imagine my return, she was now capable of bearing an absence completely unanticipated and unexplained. She was prepared to believe that others were holding her in their thoughts even when they were not present to prove it, even when they failed her.

I sat in Thirtieth Street Station across from the hot-pretzel stand and loved the feeling of the oak bench under my hands. The tall deco lamps had never burned more brightly. It was so good to be home.

•　　•　　•

Emily began to think more and more about moving to a part of the country closer to Inez, who was now in college. She started making plans to move to California, where she had made contacts through her activist friends. They offered to put her up and help her find work. It was during a discussion of her plans that she chose to evaluate her progress.

"How did therapy help me? I'm alive, first of all. No, more than that: I don't feel like a walking disaster any more. I feel like a person with good and bad points. And that I know how to love somebody."

"You made remarkable changes!" I said.

"Well, let's not flip overboard. I still smoke. I don't have a girlfriend. Sometimes I wonder if deep down you're disappointed in me. But who can say one person gets an A-minus or a C-plus in therapy?"

I didn't even bother pointing out that she had cut her smoking in half.

"'Disappointed?' Emily, therapy doesn't make people perfect. Do you remember what we decided about *change* last year—that everybody wants to feel they have learned to work and love as well as or better than their parents?"

"Yeah. We said my mother held out for me almost twice as long as her mom did for her. And I guess it's extremely cool that I gave Inez the chance to have a mom for life."

"And not just a warm body," I added, "but a mom able to listen and help her without getting in her way too much. You've given her the example of someone who can make her own life good, by going back to school and having friends. You've accomplished as much healing in one generation as some families do in five!"

Working with Emily in those final years was easy and un-traumatic. And our termination felt right as well. Winnicott compares the leaving of the "good-enough" therapist to the leaving behind of the transitional object or blanket. Once so essential to psychic safety, the blanket becomes irrelevant. It is not destroyed or eaten but, as Winnicott says, simply set aside.

• • •

Emily left Philadelphia on a rainy day in March. She sent cards from various addresses, letting me know she was doing well. My pleasure in her flourishing made certain things easier to bear—especially the death of Grace, who did not outlive us all, as I had hoped. I miss her all the time.

How do we judge the outcome of a therapy that spans one decade and a half? There are therapists who would find the outcome of my work wanting since the patient did not end up in a loving marriage or partnership. Despite the vast and rang-ing contributions made to world cultures by unmarried people, a married-is-better prejudice endures. Single women and men are pitied or scorned as immature, damaged, or selfish. Luckily, no one with this view was Emily's therapist. I was able to honor her desires, her choices, as I had those of other patients, whether to cohabit, marry, or neither.

The question of the value of marriage or constant closeness returns us to Schopenhauer's parable of the porcupines, which ends as follows:

*Wer jedoch viel eigene, innere Wärme hat, bleibt lieber aus der
Gesellschaft weg, um keine Beschwerde zu geben, noch zu empfangen.*

Those with a great deal of internal warmth preferred to stay
apart from the group, and so caused and encountered the
least trouble.

Emily was someone who had cultivated that elusive "internal warmth," allowing her both to love and to stand apart.

To choose solitude freely, to love and engage fully—both
are capacities to be desired.

Herein lies the work of the talking cure.

NOTES

Numbers preceding notes refer to pages on which corresponding text passages appear.

EPIGRAPHS

ix   "The only victory": Napoleon, *Maxims*.

ix   ". . . [T]he God of woman": M'Lissa, in A. Walker, *Possessing the Secret of Joy* (New York: Washington Square Press, 1992).

ix   "be of love": E. E. Cummings, *Complete Poems 1904–1962*, edited by G. Firmage (New York: Liveright Publishing Corporation, 1991), p. 453. Quoted with permission.

INTRODUCTION: MAKING ROOM IN LOVE FOR HATE

1   "little statues": H.D. (Hilda Doolittle), *Tribute to Freud* (New York: New Directions, 1974), p. 175.

2   "anxiety about lecturing": For the account of Freud's plan to catch sight of a porcupine *and* give lectures, see E. Jones, *Sigmund Freud: Life and Work., Vol. 2, Years of Maturity, 1901–1919* (New York: Basic Books, 1955), p. 59. Apparently, the expression "to find one's porcupine" became a recognized saying in Freud's circle.

2   "Schopenhauer's well-known fable": I am surely not the first to imagine a connection between Freud's interest in porcupines and Schopenhauer's parable. However, the only mention of such a connection I have been able to find is in an article by L. Ginsburg, "The imprint of Sigmund Freud's interest in porcupines upon the study of group constructs," *Psychoanalysis and Contemporary Thought, 8* (1985), pp. 515–528. The fable itself is in *Parerga und Paralipomena*, Vol. II (Zurich: Haffmans-Verlag, 1988), pp. 559–560. See also T. B. Saunders' translation in *The Essays of Arthur Schopenhauer* (New York: Willey Book Co., 1925), p. 100.

2–3   "group psychology": Freud discusses the Schopenhauer parable in *Group Psychology and the Analysis of the Ego* (1921), translated by J. Strachey (New York: Norton, 1959), p. 33.

3   "love/hate relations": See D. Winnicott, "Hate in the countertransference," in *Through Paediatrics to Psycho-Analysis* (New York: Basic Books, 1975), pp. 194–203.

3   "believing you are a nice person": Fay Weldon's comment is cited as a personal communication to the author in R. Parker, *Mother Love, Mother Hate* (New York: Basic Books, 1995), p. 5.

3   "There must be room in love for hate" is from Molly Peacock's poem "There Must Be," which appears in her collection *Take Heart* (New York: Vintage Books, 1989), p. 71. Quoted with permission.

7   "What is love?": Plato, *Euthyphro, Crito, Apology and Symposium* (South Bend, IN: Regnery/Gateway, 1953).

7   "I always have an anxious concern . . ." is from A. Schopenhauer, *Manuscript Remains,* Vol. 4, edited by A. Hubscher (Oxford, 1988–1990), p. 507.

7   "[T]he consolation of my life" is from *Parerga and Paralipomena,* Vol. II (Oxford: Oxford University Press, 1974), p. 397. See also C. Janaway, *Schopenhauer* (Oxford: Oxford University Press, 1994), p. 15.

7–8   Freud's relationship to Schopenhauer is complex. Upon describing his own concept of the death drive, Freud addressed his audience: "You may perhaps shrug your shoulders and say: 'That isn't natural science, it's Schopenhauer's philosophy!'" (*New Introductory Lectures* [New York: Norton], p. 95). Freud insisted elsewhere that he had not even read Schopenhauer until late in life. However, since every educated European of that time would have had some acquaintance with the philosopher's work, there is no reason to conclude that Freud could *not* have had Schopenhauer's porcupines in mind when he made his trip to America in 1909, even though he didn't cite the fable until 1921 in *Group Psychology.* For more on the relationship between these two thinkers, see C. Young and A. Brook, "Schopenhauer and Freud," *International Journal of Psycho-Analysis, 75* (February 1994), pp. 101–118.

8   "Anna O." was the pseudonym given to activist and feminist Bertha Pappenheim, history's first psychoanalytic patient. See J. Breuer and S. Freud, *Studies on Hysteria* (New York: Basic Books, 1982), pp. 21–47. For a discussion of Pappenheim's career, see L. Appignanesi and J. Forrester, *Freud's Women* (New York: Basic Books, 1992).

8   "underlying psychology": B. Spock, *Baby and Child Care* (New York: Pocket Books, 1998), p. 33. This book has sold over 50 million copies.

8   "a whole climate of opinion": W. H. Auden, "In Memory of Sigmund Freud," in *Collected Poems,* edited by E. Mendelson (New York: Vintage Books, 1991), p. 275.

8   "on the couch": S. Caesar (as told to R. Gehman), "What psychoanalysis did for me," *Look* (October 2, 1956), pp. 48–51.

8   "One in ten Americans have taken Prozac": See J. Glenmullen, *Prozac Backlash* (New York: Simon & Schuster, 2000), p. 15. See also P. Breggin, *Talking Back to Ritalin: What Doctors Aren't Telling You About Stimulants and ADHD* (Cambridge, MA: Perseus, 2001).

9   "psychotherapy alters our brain chemistry": Psychiatrist Susan Vaughan describes research suggesting that therapy elevates serotonin levels. See her *The Talking Cure* (New York: Henry Holt, 1997).

9   "I am a psychoanalyst": R. Lindner, *The Fifty-Minute Hour* (New York: Rinehart & Co., 1954). Lindner is probably best known as the author of *Rebel Without a Cause*.

10   "the use of the countertransference": S. Orbach, *The Impossibility of Sex* (New York: Viking, 2000).

10   "no perfect solution to the problem of writing": See the issue of *Psychoanalytic Dialogues—10*, no. 2 (2000)—dedicated to the ethical and clinical complexities of this problem.

10–11   "no one mistaking wife for hat": See O. Sacks, *The Man Who Mistook His Wife for a Hat* (New York: Harper & Row, 1987).

11   "case histories fictional": P. Roth, *My Life as a Man* (New York: Vintage Books, 1970), p. 242.

12   "transference and resistance": See S. Freud, *On the History of the Psycho-Analytic Movement* (1914) (New York: Norton, 1966), p. 16.

12   "the transference relationship": For Freud's view of countertransference, see his "The future prospects of psychoanalytic therapy," in *Therapy and Technique* (New York: Norton, 1963), pp. 80–81. For a contemporary view of the countertransference as a valuable instrument of the treatment, see M. Tansey and W. Burke, *Understanding Countertransference* (Hillsdale, NJ: Analytic Press, 1989). See also A. Green, *On Private Madness* (Madison, CT: International Universities Press, 1972).

14   "a third essential element": For Winnicott's views of play and of holding in psychoanalysis, see his *Playing and Reality* (London: Tavistock Publications, 1971) and *Home Is Where We Start From* (New York: Norton, 1986).

14   "the good-enough mother": "'The good mother' and 'the bad mother' of the Kleinian jargon are internal objects and are nothing to do with real women. The best a real woman can do with an infant is to be sensitively good *enough*. . . . " See D. Winnicott in *The Spontaneous Gesture*, edited by F. Rodman (Cambridge, MA: Harvard University Press, 1987), p. 38.

15   "The cipher of his mortal destiny" is a phrase from J. Lacan, "The mirror stage as formative of the function of the I," in *Écrits*, translated by A. Sheridan (New York: Norton, 1977), p. 7.

15   "understand three (not just two) generations": The importance placed on three generations emerges in Lacan's seminar on the transference (not yet translated into English). See *Le séminaire, Livre VIII, Le transfert* (1960–1961) (Paris: Seuil, 1991).

15   "The sexual relationship does not exist": This concept is described in J. Lacan, *Encore: The Seminar of Jacques Lacan, Book XX*, translated by B. Fink (New York: Norton, 1999), p. 66.

15   Lacan discusses the *Symposium* and criticizes Aristophanic love in his *Le transfert*.

16 "the goals of analysis": Lacanians do not see analysis as "therapeutic" and thus might derive support from Freud's remark that "[m]y discoveries are not primarily a heal-all. My discoveries are a basis for a very grave philosophy. There are very few who understand this." Quoted in H.D. (Hilda Doolittle), *Tribute to Freud* (New York: New Directions, 1974), p. 18. For clinical case examples of Lacanian psychoanalysis, see S. Schneiderman, *Returning to Freud* (New Haven: Yale University Press, 1980).

16 "Winnicott had no contempt for therapy": Indeed, he did not view its aims as contrary to those of psychoanalysis. See Freud's essay "On psychotherapy," in *Therapy and Technique* (1904) (New York: Collier Books, 1963), pp. 63–76.

19 "the porcupine dilemmas of everyday life": Here, I am paraphrasing a well-known Freudian remark: "[M]uch will be gained if we succeed in transforming your hysterical misery into common unhappiness." In J. Breuer and S. Freud, *Studies on Hysteria* (New York: Basic Books, 1982), p. 305.

CHAPTER 1: SAME BED, DIFFERENT DREAMS

21 "Every marriage is really two": J. Bernard, *The Future of Marriage* (New York: Bantam Books, 1972).

21 "Same bed, different dreams": As I understand it, the Chinese version, *tong chuang yi meng*, implies a married couple living together with different agendas.

29 "exchange of emotions": The term "projective identification" was coined by Melanie Klein to describe the infant's splitting off unbearable affects and "storing" them in the mother's breast. Object relations theorists have extended its use to other relationships. See M. Tansey and W. Burke, *Understanding Countertransference: From Projective Identification to Empathy*. The term should not be confused with simple "projection," which does not imply that another person has taken on the split-off emotions.

43 "family in crisis": Leroy Johnson's story is told in D. Luepnitz, *The Family Interpreted* (New York: Basic Books, 1988), pp. 280–316.

46 "Nobody ever eats alone": See C. Bloom et al., *Eating Problems* (New York: Basic Books, 1994).

49 "wounded self-esteem": R. Sennett and J. Cobb, *The Hidden Injuries of Class* (New York: Norton, 1972).

52 Lacan's use of "castration" is different from the conventional sexist usage, which implies that women, who are supposed to be weak, try to "castrate" men, who are supposed to be strong. Biological masculinity and femininity are not at stake in Lacan's usage. He writes: "The woman has to undergo no more or less castration than the man." See *Seminar of 21 January 1975*, edited by J. Mitchell and J. Rose, in *Feminine Sexuality* (New York: Norton, 1982), p. 168.

60 "They were projecting their anxieties onto Rosie": This was simple projection. It would have become projective identification only if they had

managed to store their fears in the child. She was not acting afraid at that point—they were.

CHAPTER 2: CHRISTMAS IN JULY

66   "Superlabile diabetic" is a term that was used routinely by researchers and clinicians at the Philadelphia Child Guidance Clinic in the 1980s to refer to diabetics whose condition was governed by psychosomatic factors. See S. Minuchin, *Families and Family Therapy* (Cambridge, MA: Harvard University Press, 1974), p. 7. Diabetic science has greatly advanced since then.

68   "research on children's psychosomatic disorders": See S. Minuchin, B. Rosman, and L. Baker, *Psychosomatic Families* (Cambridge, MA: Harvard University Press, 1978).

79   "Give me another family": This is the kind of parapraxis that Freud describes in *The Psychopathology of Everyday Life* (1901) (New York: Norton, 1960).

80   "This family plan . . ." is in S. Freud, "Notes upon a case of an obsessional neurosis," in *Three Case Histories* (1909) (New York: Collier Books, 1963), pp. 56–57.

85   "Squiggles": See D. Winnicott, "The Squiggle Game," in *Psychoanalytic Explorations* (Cambridge, MA: Harvard University Press, 1989), pp. 299–317.

90   "If I am not for myself . . . ": *Pirke Avot*, Vol. 1, p. 14.

92   "This is the age when": C. Gilligan, *In a Different Voice* (Cambridge, MA: Harvard University Press, 1982). See also *The Birth of Pleasure* (forthcoming).

99   "three registers": Lacan's concept of the three registers appears in his first seminar and is developed throughout the course of his work. See *The Seminar of Jacques Lacan, Book I, 1953–4*, translated by J. Forrester (New York: Norton, 1988). For a good introduction to the three registers, see R. Samuels, *Between Philosophy and Psychoanalysis* (New York: Routledge, 1993).

100   "potential space": See D. Winnicott, *Playing and Reality* (London: Tavistock, 1971).

101   The story of the Good Samaritan is found in Luke 10:30–35.

CHAPTER 3: DON JUAN IN TRENTON

105   "uncanny . . . in the Freudian sense": See S. Freud, "The uncanny" (1919), in *Studies in Parapsychology* (New York: Collier, 1963), pp. 19–62.

109   "'false self' or 'as if' personality": "False self" is Winnicott's term, whereas "'as if' personality" originated with H. Deutsch (see "Some forms of emotional disturbances and their relationship to schizophrenia," in *Neuroses and Character Types* [New York: International Universities Press, 1965]) and was adopted by M. Khan (*The Privacy of the Self* [London: Hogarth, 1974]).

109   "true self goes into cold storage": D. Winnicott, "Mirror role of mother and family in child development," in *Playing and Reality* (London: Routledge, 1971), pp. 111–118.

109   *El Burlador de Sevilla y el convidado de piedra*, translated by G. Edwards (Warminster, UK: Aris & Phillips, 1986). *Burlador* means "trickster."

110   O. Rank, *The Don Juan Legend*, translated by D. Winter (Princeton, NJ: Princeton University Press, 1975), p. 41; originally published in 1930.

111   "terrible Argentine movie": My reference here is to *The Dark Side of the Heart.*

115   "King Nebuchadnezzar": The king says to a group of servants, "The thing is gone from me: if ye will not make known unto me the dream, with the interpretation thereof, ye shall be cut in pieces, and your houses shall be made a dunghill" (Daniel 2:3–6). Daniel prevails by asking for more time.

118   "with women he was what . . . ": G. Byron, *Don Juan* (New York: Penguin, 1973), Canto XV, 16, p. 501.

121   "Something deadening happens to boys": C. Gilligan, *The Birth of Pleasure* (forthcoming).

122   "refusing to be a man": J. Stoltenberg, *Refusing to Be a Man* (Portland, OR: Breitenbush Books, 1989).

129   "depression as an achievement": Here, Winnicott was building on Melanie Klein's work, which describes the infant's depressive position as a developmental stage beyond the early paranoid-schizoid position. See D. Winnicott, "The value of depression," in *Home Is Where We Start From*, edited by C. Winnicott (New York: Basic Books, 1986), pp. 71–79.

132   "anti-abortion people who become *de facto* pro-choice": Clinic workers who endure daily attacks by anti-choice fanatics have wrestled with the question of whether to provide abortions to those very women when they come in as clients. The Allentown Women's Center in Pennsylvania faced this problem and asked such women, as a condition for obtaining an abortion, to sign a paper stating that the procedure should remain legal. NOW's then-president Molly Yard opposed the move, saying the clinic should offer its services to all women, unconditionally. See "Testing patients' politics: Clinic puts conditions on abortion foes," *Philadelphia Inquirer*, August 2, 1989.

132   "the compulsion to repeat": See S. Freud, *Beyond the Pleasure Principle* (1922) (New York: Norton, 1961).

141   "that woman's face": Karen Horney's essay "The dread of woman" (in *Feminine Psychology* [New York: Norton, 1967], pp. 133–146) describes men's primitive contempt for women as a reaction formation against their own feelings of inferiority. The little boy desires his mother, but also fears his body is inadequate to please her. Instead of experiencing himself as small and vulnerable, he sees the mother as huge, devouring, dangerous. In a similar vein, note that powerful and unruly aspects of nature are often feminized. See also D. Dinnerstein, *The Mermaid and the Minotaur* (New York: Harper & Row, 1976).

148   "political topics in the consulting room": A. Samuels, *The Political Psyche* (London: Routledge, 1993). See also *Politics on the Couch* (New York: Other Press, 2001).

149   "throwing out the Oedipus complex": See G. Deleuze and F. Guattari, *Anti-Oedipus* (New York: Viking, 1977), in which the authors, romanticizing madness, aim to replace psychoanalysis with "schizoanalysis." Feminist critiques of Oedipal thinking include L. Irigaray, *Speculum of the Other Woman* (Ithaca, NY: Cornell University Press, 1985), and C. Gilligan, *The Birth of Pleasure* (forthcoming). Gilligan suggests that we replace the Oedipus myth with that of Eros and Psyche, not only because its protagonist is female but also because it ends with marriage and the birth of a daughter rather than with death and loss. N. O'Connor and J. Ryan don't want to eliminate Oedipal theory as much as they want to make it less coercive and narrow. See their *Wild Desires and Mistaken Identities: Lesbianism and Psychoanalysis* (New York: Columbia University Press, 1993). For a critique of Oedipus that focuses on issues of culture and race, see F. Fanon, *Black Skin, White Masks* (New York: Grove Press, 1967). See also C. Bollas, "Why Oedipus?" in *Being a Character* (New York: Hill & Wang, 1992). Lacan maintained that the Oedipus complex was the cornerstone of psychoanalysis, but added a fourth term to the conventional triad of mother, father, child—namely, death. He felt that Sophocles' *Oedipus at Colonus* held more for analysts than *Oedipus Rex*. See J. Lacan, "The neurotic's individual myth," translated by M. Evans, *Psychoanalytic Quarterly, 48* (1979), pp. 405–425.

CHAPTER 4: A DARWINIAN FINCH

150   "What a trifling difference": C. Darwin, letter to Asa Gray, in *The Correspondence of Charles Darwin*, 8 vols., edited by F. Burkhardt and S. Smith (Cambridge, UK: Cambridge University Press, 1985).

155   *"the manic defense"*: See M. Klein, "On the theory of anxiety and guilt," in *Envy and Gratitude* (London: Hogarth Press, 1975), pp. 25–42.

157   "feminists have pointed out": See, for example, L. Eichenbaum and S. Orbach, *Understanding Women: A Feminist Psychoanalytic View* (New York: Basic Books, 1983).

158   "the sound of my own voice": J. Kincaid, *Annie John* (New York: Noonday Press, 1983), p. 41.

159   *"impingements"*: D. Winnicott, *Psychoanalytic Explorations* (Cambridge, MA: Harvard University Press, 1989).

161   "Self psychologists": See H. Kohut, *The Analysis of the Self* (New York: International Universities Press, 1971).

161   "ability to *recognize* her infant": see D. Winnicott, "Mirror role of mother and family in child development," in *Playing and Reality* (London: Routledge, 1971), pp. 111–118.

161   "mirror phase": See J. Lacan, "The mirror stage as formative of the function of the I as revealed in psychoanalytic experience," in *Écrits*, translated by A. Sheridan (New York: Norton, 1977), pp. 1–7.

161 "reflecting the figure of man": See V. Woolf, *A Room of One's Own* (New York: Harcourt, Brace & World, 1929), p. 35.

167 "*such a paradise*": J. Kincaid, *Annie John*, p. 25 (emphasis added).

167 "nothing in nature more powerful than the maternal instinct": Darwin says, for example, "But the most curious instance known to me of one instinct conquering another, is the migratory instinct conquering the maternal instinct. . . . The former is wonderfully strong. . . . Nevertheless, the migratory instinct is so powerful that late in the autumn swallows and housemartins frequently desert their tender young, leaving them to perish miserably in their nests." See *The Descent of Man* (Princeton, NJ: Princeton University Press, 1981), pp. 83–84.

169 "Delaney sisters": See S. Delaney and A. Delaney, *Having Our Say* (New York: Dell, 1993).

169 "termination of analysis": See M. Klein, "On the criteria for the termination of a psycho-analysis," in *Envy and Gratitude*, p. 45. Klein's goal here is to describe the reduction of depressive and persecutory anxiety as ends of analysis; she is not discussing sexuality. However, the fact that she could so casually add heterosexuality as a criterion suggests that much had already been done to bowdlerize Freud. Freud not only stated that homosexuality was not an illness, he also vehemently disagreed with Jones and others about barring homosexual men and women as analysts. See M. Magee and D. Miller, *Lesbian Lives: Psychoanalytic Narratives Old and New* (Hillsdale, NJ: Analytic Press, 1997).

170 "Many abused girls say just that": See J. Herman, *Father-Daughter Incest* (Cambridge, MA: Harvard University Press, 1981).

171 "many people repress traumatic events": See the excellent study by L. Williams in which 129 women with histories of sexual abuse as girls were asked about their abuse histories. Fully 38 percent of these women did not recall the events documented seventeen years earlier. Those who had been molested at the youngest ages and those molested by someone they knew were least likely to remember the events. See "Recall of childhood trauma: A prospective study of women's memories of child sexual abuse," *Journal of Consulting and Clinical Psychology, 62* (1994), pp. 1167–1176.

173 "The key to our conundrum lay in an article": F. Sulloway, "Darwin and his finches: The evolution of a legend," *Journal of the History of Biology, 15* (1982), pp. 1–53. The quotation is on p. 40.

174 "careful not to interbreed": D. Lack, *Darwin's Finches*, edited by L. Ratcliffe and P. Boag (Cambridge, UK: Cambridge University Press, 1983).

174 "the most robust of all": See P. Grant and R. Grant, "Hybridization of bird species," *Science, 256* (1992), pp. 193–197. See also J. Weiner's beautiful *The Beak of the Finch* (New York: Vintage, 1994). According to Weiner, although Darwin did not know about the existence of genes and the genetic

code, he predicted their discovery. He imagined them as a "swarm of letters streaming through the blood." Darwin wrote: "And these characters, like those written on paper with invisible ink, lie ready to be evolved whenever the organisation is disturbed by certain known or unknown conditions" (p. 214). Darwin here is a proto-Lacanian, concerned with the relationship between the letter and the real.

177   "the register of the symbolic": The importance of the symbolic register is highlighted in J. Lacan, "The function and field of speech and language in psychoanalysis," in *Écrits*, translated by A. Sheridan (New York: Norton, 1977), pp. 30–113. His attention to the impact of family names is evident in his seminar on the transference in the discussion of Claudel's "Coûfontaine family." See *Le séminaire, Livre VIII* (Paris: Seuil, 1991).

177   "Even before we speak": See J. Lacan, *The Seminar of Jacques Lacan, Book II: The Ego in Freud's Theory and in the Technique of Psychoanalysis* (1954–1955), translated by Sylvana Tomaselli (New York: Norton, 1988).

178   "a more lasting grace than beauty": Sophocles, *Oedipus at Colonus,* in *Complete Greek Tragedies*, Vol. 1, edited by D. Greene and R. Lattimore, translated by D. Greene (Chicago: University of Chicago Press, 1954), scene 3, p. 105.

185   "Those wrecked by success" is part of an essay titled "Some character types met with in psychoanalytic work," in S. Freud, *Character and Culture* (1916) (New York: Collier, 1963), pp. 157–181. Both quotations are found on pp. 162–163.

186   I first encountered the term "frozen grief" in the work of psychoanalyst Marie Langer, who lived and worked in Nicaragua during the revolution. Her biographer, Nancy Hollander, writes that "[Langer] spoke of the widespread phenomenon in Nicaragua of what she called 'frozen grief.' She explained that a large number of individuals have experienced losses in the revolutionary struggle and the Contra war and have not had the opportunity . . . to mourn. She pointed out that a person who has not grieved the loss of loved ones may suffer apparently unrelated symptoms, such as psychosomatic illnesses or interpersonal conflicts. The person . . . remains fixed in the past." See M. Langer, *From Vienna to Managua: Journey of a Psychoanalyst*, translated by M. Hooks (London: Free Association Books, 1989), p. 6.

187   "mourning over lost time": S. Freud, "Mourning and melancholia," in *General Psychological Theory* (1917) (New York: Collier, 1963), pp. 164–179.

189   "In the tendency of mothers to overidentify": S. Freud, "Female sexuality," in *Sexuality and the Psychology of Love* (1931) (New York: Collier, 1963), pp. 194–211.

189   "the difference between boys and girls": Chodorow follows Freud's explanation of the nature of mothers' attachment to girls and boys, but argues for different implications. See N. Chodorow, *The Reproduction of Mothering* (Berkeley: University of California Press, 1978).

190   "Something I could not name": J. Kincaid, *Annie John*, p. 88.

193   "Race matters": *Race Matters* is the title of a wonderful book by Cornel West (Boston: Beacon Press, 1993).

194   "rather than disavow one's own resistances": In the intervening years, I have come to think that another aspect of my resistance was deciding very early on that there could be "no comparison" between our backgrounds since I am white and had not known grinding poverty. It felt self-indulgent to compare my lot as a child with hers—but the fact is, there were correspondences, and I did experience a strong affinity with her. Just as one can overplay identifications and assume one can feel the other's pain, so is it also possible to shrink from these thoughts too soon. Philip Cushman has said that being "white" in this society means having money and power, and whites who don't are, to some degree, merely "passing" as white. One could say that I resisted remembering my own marginality and class-related humiliations, and was thus allowing Pearl to contain them for me. Making her the poor black woman meant I could be truly white! I owe these reflections to two recent articles: P. Cushman, "White guilt, political activity and the analyst," *Psychoanalytic Dialogues, 10* (2000), pp. 607–618, and J. Gump, "A white therapist, an African-American patient—Shame in the therapeutic dyad," *Psychoanalytic Dialogues, 10* (2000), pp. 619–632.

194   "black enough": K. Leary, "Racial enactments in dynamic treatment," in *Psychoanalytic Dialogues, 10* (2000), pp. 639–654.

CHAPTER 5: THE SIN EATER

201   "*whole families live here*": The inpatient service of our clinic maintained two apartments where families in crisis (most, but not all poor) would live for up to two months, receiving round-the-clock services. Afterward, they were assigned an outpatient therapist. This remarkable, world-famous program was eliminated in the first round of budget cuts.

201   "20 percent work full time": This is a Project H.O.M.E. statistic. A U.S. Department of Housing and Urban Development report in 1999 found that 44 percent of homeless adults work at least part time. See M. Otto, "44% of homeless people have jobs, HUD reports," *Philadelphia Inquirer*, December 21, 1999, p. A21.

205   "The name [Emily] came to me" not as a pseudonym for *Schopenhauer's Porcupines*, obviously, but simply as a description of my experience of my patient. See D. Lessing, *Memoirs of a Survivor* (New York: Knopf, 1975).

213   "borderline personality": Among those who have contributed to the definition and treatment of borderline conditions are J. Masterson, *Psychotherapy of the Borderline Adult* (New York: Brunner/Mazel, 1976), and O. Kernberg, *Object Relations Theory and Clinical Psychoanalysis* (New York: Jason Aronson, 1976). For works by young women diagnosed as borderline, see E. Gordon, *Mockingbird Years* (New York: Basic Books, 2000), and S. Kaysen,

Girl, Interrupted (New York: Vintage, 1993). For a brilliant critique of the borderline diagnosis and its politics, see M. Layton, "Emerging from the shadows," *Networker*, May–June (1995), pp. 35–41. See also J. Davies and M. Frawley, *Treating the Adult Survivor of Childhood Sexual Abuse: A Psychoanalytic Perspective* (New York: Basic Books, 1994).

214   "Winnicott's classic paper": See D. Winnicott, "Hate in the countertransference," in *Through Paediatrics to Psycho-Analysis* (New York: Basic Books, 1975).

218   "I am alive": E. Dickinson, *The Complete Poems of Emily Dickinson*, Poem #470, edited by T. Johnson (Boston: Little, Brown & Co., 1960), pp. 225–226.

222   "a conversation about symptomatic eating": See K. Chernin, *The Obsession* (New York: Harper & Row, 1981), and C. Bloom et al., *Eating Problems* (New York: Basic Books, 1994).

224   "Disgusting Matt," in addition to referring to the trauma with her uncle, could refer to the primitive, pre-Oedipal terrors that Lacan described with the concept of *das Ding*. See *The Seminar of Jacques Lacan. Book VII, The Ethics of Psychoanalysis 1959–60*, translated by D. Porter (New York: Norton, 1992).

224   "one girl in six": See J. Herman, *Father-Daughter Incest* (Cambridge, MA: Harvard University Press, 1981).

233   "Do you remember me telling you": Sin eating was practiced in Wales through the nineteenth century, and also in Appalachia where a number of Welsh immigrants settled. The food placed on the corpse was salted bread—not the full feast represented in the television show. My information comes from Mr. Robin Gwyndaf, director of the Museum of Welsh Life in Cardiff, Wales. The practice is mentioned in many novels and short stories, including M. Webb's *Precious Bane* and M. Atwood's "The Sin Eater" in *Dancing Girls and Other Stories* (New York: Simon & Schuster, 1982).

235   "a group estimated to number 3.6 million": D. Morrow, "Lusting after Prozac," *New York Times*, October 11, 1998, section 3, p. 1.

237   "sexuality is never 'one thing'": For example, in 1899, Freud wrote to Fliess, "But bisexuality! You are certainly right about it. I am accustoming myself to regarding every sexual act as a process in which four individuals are involved." See *The Complete Letters of Sigmund Freud to Wilhelm Fliess*, translated by J. Masson (Cambridge, MA: Harvard University Press, 1985), p. 364.

237   "Little Hans": S. Freud, "Analysis of a phobia in a five-year-old boy" (1909), in *The Sexual Enlightenment of Children* (New York: Collier, 1963), pp. 47–184.

238   "two aspects of the complex, the positive and negative": S. Freud, *The Ego and the Id* (New York: Norton, 1962), p. 23.

238   "capable of making a homosexual object-choice": S. Freud, *Three Essays on the Theory of Sexuality* (New York: Basic Books, 1962), p. 11.

238   "Homosexuality . . . cannot be classified as an illness": S. Freud, *The Letters of Sigmund Freud*, edited by E. Freud (New York: Basic Books, 1960); letter of April 9, 1935, p. 277.

239   "classified homosexuality as a pathological condition until 1973": An excellent source on this issue is *Homosexuality and Psychoanalysis*, edited by T. Dean and C. Lane (Chicago: University of Chicago Press, 2001).

239   "Books on sexuality by psychoanalysts who are themselves gay or lesbian": See K. Lewes, *The Psychoanalytic Theory of Male Homosexuality* (New York: New American Library, 1988), and M. Magee and D. Miller, *Lesbian Lives: Psychoanalytic Narratives Old and New* (Hillsdale, NJ: Analytic Press, 1997).

239   "full bisexuality": K. Chernin, *A Different Kind of Listening* (New York: HarperCollins, 1995).

248   "Single women and men are pitied": M. Clements, *The Improvised Woman: Single Women Re-inventing Single Life* (New York: Norton, 1998).

249   "*Wer jedoch viel eigene*": A. Schopenhauer, *Parerga und Paralipomena*, Vol. II (Zurich: Haffmans-Verlag, 1988), pp. 559–560.

249   "Those with a great deal of internal warmth": This is my own translation, which I prefer to the standard renderings because they introduce the word "man" or "his," which do not exist in the original.

BIBLIOGRAPHY

Appignanesi, L., and Forrester, J. (1992). *Freud's Women*. New York: Basic Books.

Aron, L. (1995). "The internalized primal scene." *Psychoanalytic Dialogues, 5*, pp. 195–238.

Benjamin, J. (1988). *The Bonds of Love*. New York: Pantheon.

_____. (1995). *Like Subjects, Love Objects*. New Haven: Yale University Press.

Bernard, J. (1972). *The Future of Marriage*. New York: Bantam Books.

Bloom, C., Gitter, A., Gutwill, S., Kogel, L., and Zaphiropoulos, L. (1994). *Eating Problems: A Feminist Psychoanalytic Treatment Model*. New York: Basic Books.

Bollas, C. (1992). *Being a Character: Psychoanalysis and Self Experience*. New York: Hill and Wang.

Bracher, M. (1993). *Lacan, Discourse, and Social Change*. Ithaca, NY: Cornell University Press.

Breggin, P. (2001). *Talking Back to Ritalin: What Doctors Aren't Telling You About Stimulants and ADHD*. Cambridge, MA: Perseus, 2001.

Breuer, J., and Freud, S. (1982). *Studies on Hysteria*. New York: Basic Books.

Byron, G. (1977). *Don Juan*, edited by T. Steffan, E. Steffan, and W. Pratt. London: Penguin Books.

Chernin, K. (1981). *The Obsession*. New York: Harper & Row.

_____. (1995). *A Different Kind of Listening*. New York: HarperCollins.

Chodorow, N. (1978). *The Reproduction of Mothering*. Berkeley: University of California Press.

Clements, M. (1998). *The Improvised Woman: Single Women Re-inventing Single Life*. New York: Norton.

Conway, K. (1997). *Ordinary Life: A Memoir of Illness*. New York: W. H. Freeman & Co.

Coontz, S. (1992). *The Way We Never Were*. New York: Basic Books.

Corbett, K. (2001). "More life: Centrality and marginality in human development." *Psychoanalytic Dialogues, 11*, pp. 313–335.

Cummings, E. E. (1991). *Complete Poems, 1904–1962*, edited by G. Firmage. New York: Liveright Publishing Corporation.

Darwin, C. (1839/1987). *Diary of the Voyage of the H.M.S. Beagle, Vol. 1, The Works of Charles Darwin*, edited by P. Barnett and P. Freeman. New York: New York University Press.

_____. (1859/1964). *On the Origin of Species*, edited by E. Mayr. Cambridge, MA: Harvard University Press.

———. (1871/1981). *The Descent of Man, and Selection in Relation to Sex.* Princeton, NJ: Princeton University Press.

Davis, A. (1983). *Women, Race, and Class.* New York: Vintage.

———. (1998). *Blues Legacies and Black Feminism.* New York: Pantheon.

Dean, T., and Lane, C. (2001). *Homosexuality and Psychoanalysis.* Chicago: University of Chicago Press.

De Botton, A. (1997). *How Proust Can Change Your Life.* New York: Vintage.

Dickinson, E. (1960). *The Complete Poems of Emily Dickinson,* edited by T. Johnson. Boston: Little, Brown & Co.

Dimen, M. (1994). "Money, love, and hate: Contradiction and paradox." *Psychoanalytic Dialogues, 4,* pp. 69–100.

Dinnerstein, D. (1976). *The Mermaid and the Minotaur: Sexual Arrangements and Human Malaise.* New York: Harper & Row.

Ehrenreich, B. (1983). *The Hearts of Men.* Garden City, NY: Doubleday.

Eichenbaum, L., and Orbach, S. (1983). *Understanding Women: A Feminist Psychoanalytic View.*

Epstein, M. (1995). *Thoughts Without a Thinker.* New York: Basic Books.

Falkenheim, J. (1993). "The education of a clinical social worker: Finding a place for the humanities." *Clinical Social Work Journal, 21,* pp. 85–96.

Fanon, F. (1967). *Black Skin, White Masks.* New York: Grove Press.

———. (1968). The *Wretched of the Earth,* translated by C. Farrington. New York: Grove Press.

Felman, S. (1987). *Jacques Lacan and the Adventure of Insight.* Cambridge, MA: Harvard University Press.

Forrester, J. (1990). *The Seductions of Psychoanalysis.* Cambridge, UK: Cambridge University Press.

———. (1997). *Dispatches from the Freud Wars.* Cambridge, MA: Harvard University Press.

Foucault, M. (1978). *The History of Sexuality,* Vol. 1, translated by R. Hurley. York: Random House.

Freud, E. (1960). *The Letters of Sigmund Freud,* translated by T. Stern and J. Stern. London: Hogarth Press.

Freud, S. (1961). *The Standard Edition of the Complete Psychological Works of Sigmund Freud,* 24 vols., translated by J. Strachey. London: Hogarth Press.

Gerson, M. (1996). *The Embedded Self: A Psychoanalytic Guide to Family Therapy.* Hillsdale, NJ: Analytic Press.

Gilbert, L. (2002). *The Last American Man.* New York: Viking.

Gilligan, C. (1982). *In a Different Voice.* Cambridge, MA: Harvard University Press.

Gilman, S. (1993). *Freud, Race, and Gender.* Princeton, NJ: Princeton University Press.

Glenmullen, J. (2000). *Prozac Backlash.* New York: Simon & Schuster.

Goldner, V. (1991). "Toward a critical relational theory of gender." *Psychoanalytic Dialogues, 1,* pp. 243–248.

Green, A. (1972). *On Private Madness*. Madison, CT: International Universities Press.

Greenberg, J. (1991). *Oedipus and Beyond: A Clinical Theory*. Cambridge, MA: Harvard University Press.

Greenberg, J., and Mitchell, S. (1983). *Object Relations in Psychoanalytic Theory*. Cambridge, MA: Harvard University Press.

Greer, G. (1991). *The Change: Women, Aging, and Menopause*. New York: Ballantine.

Gump, J. (2000). "A white therapist, an African-American patient—Shame in the therapeutic dyad." *Psychoanalytic Dialogues, 10*, pp. 619–633.

H.D. (Hilda Doolittle) (1974). *Tribute to Freud*. New York: New Directions.

Herman, J. (1981). *Father-Daughter Incest*. Cambridge, MA: Harvard University Press.

———. (1992). *Trauma and Recovery*. New York: Basic Books.

Hollander, N. (1989). *From Vienna to Managua: Journey of a Psychoanalyst*. London: Free Association Books.

———. (1997). *Love in a Time of Hate: Liberation Psychology in Latin America*. New Brunswick, NJ: Rutgers University Press.

hooks, b. (2000). *All About Love*. New York: William Morrow.

Horney, K. (1967). *Feminine Psychology*. New York: Norton.

Jacoby, R. (1975). *Social Amnesia*. Boston: Beacon Press.

———. (1983). *The Repression of Psychoanalysis*. New York: Basic Books.

Janaway, C. (1994). *Schopenhauer*. New York: Oxford University Press.

Kincaid, J. (1983). *Annie John*. New York: Farrar, Straus & Giroux.

———. (1990). *Lucy*. New York: Penguin.

———. (1996). *The Autobiography of My Mother*. New York: Penguin.

Klein, M. (1975). *Envy and Gratitude and Other Works 1946–1963*. London: Hogarth.

Kovel, J. (1970). *White Racism: A Psychohistory*. New York: Pantheon.

Kramer, P. (1989). *Moments of Engagement*. New York: Penguin.

———. (1993). *Listening to Prozac*. New York: Viking.

Lacan, J. (1938/1988). *Les complexes familiaux dans la formation de l'individu*. Paris: Navarin. Translated by C. Asp in abridged form under the title "The family complexes," *Critical Texts, 5*, pp. 12–29.

———. (1977). *Écrits: A selection*, translated by A. Sheridan. New York: Norton.

———. (1979). "The neurotic's individual myth." *Psychoanalytic Quarterly, 48*, pp. 405–425.

———. (1988a). *The Seminar of Jacques Lacan. Book I, 1953–54. Freud's Papers on Technique*, translated by J. Forrester. New York: Norton.

———. (1988b). *The Seminar of Jacques Lacan. Book II, The Ego in Freud's Theory and in the Technique of Psychoanalysis* (1954–1955), translated by S. Tomaselli. New York: Norton.

———. (1988c). Seminar on "The Purloined Letter," translated by J. Mehlman. In *The Purloined Poe: Lacan, Derrida, and Psychoanalytic Reading*, edited by J. Muller and W. Richardson. Baltimore: Johns Hopkins University Press.

_____. (1991). *Le séminaire. Livre VIII, Le transfert*, edited by J. Miller. Paris: Seuil.

_____. (1992). *The Seminar of Jacques Lacan. Book VII, The Ethics of Psychoanalysis* (1959–1960), translated by D. Porter. New York: Norton.

_____. (1993). *The Seminar of Jacques Lacan. Book III, The Psychoses* (1955–1956), translated by R. Grigg. New York: Norton.

_____. (1994). *Le séminaire. Livre IV, La relation d'objet*, edited by J. Miller. Paris: Seuil.

_____. (1998). *The Seminar of Jacques Lacan. Book XX, Encore: Feminine Sexuality: The Limits of Love and Knowledge* (1972–1973), translated by B. Fink. New York: Norton.

Langer, M. (1992). *Motherhood and Sexuality*, translated by N. Hollander. New York: Guilford.

Laplanche, J., and Pontalis, J. B. (1973). *The Language of Psychoanalysis*, translated by D. Nicholson-Smith. New York: Norton.

Layton, M. (1995). "Emerging from the shadows: Looking beyond the borderline diagnosis." *Family Therapy Networker* (May/June), pp. 35–41.

Lear, J. (1998). *Open Minded*. Cambridge, MA: Harvard University Press.

Leary, K. (2000). "Racial enactments in dynamic treatment." *Psychoanalytic Dialogues, 10,* pp. 639–655.

Leclaire, S. (1971). *Démasquer le réel*. Paris: Seuil.

Lerner, H. (1988). *Women in Therapy*. New York: Jason Aronson.

Lessing, D. (1975). *Memoirs of a Survivor*. New York: Knopf.

Liebow, E.(1995). *Tell Them Who I Am: The Lives of Homeless Women*. New York: Penguin.

Lindner, R. (1954). *The Fifty-Minute Hour*. New York: Bantam.

Lippmann, P. (1996). "On dreams and interpersonal psychoanalysis." *Psychoanalytic Dialogues, 6,* pp. 831–846.

Luepnitz, D. (1988). *The Family Interpreted: Psychoanalysis, Feminism, and Family Therapy*. New York: Basic Books.

_____. (1996). "'I want you to be a woman': Reading desire in Stoller's case of 'Mrs. G.'" *Clinical Studies: International Journal of Psychoanalysis, 2,* pp. 49–58.

_____. (2002). "The phallus and beyond: Lacan, feminism, and analysis." In J.-M. Rabaté, (ed.) *The Cambridge Companion to Lacan*. Cambridge, U.K.: Cambridge University Press.

Magee, M., and Miller, D. (1997). *Lesbian Lives: Psychoanalytic Narratives Old and New*. Hillsdale, NJ: Analytic Press.

Malcolm, J. (1980). *Psychoanalysis: The Impossible Profession*. New York: Vintage.

Miller, A. (1983). *For Your Own Good*. New York: Farrar, Straus & Giroux.

Mitchell, J. (1974). *Psychoanalysis and Feminism*. New York: Vintage.

Mitchell, J., and Rose, J. (1985). *Feminine Sexuality: Jacques Lacan and the École Freudienne*. New York: Norton.

Molière, J. B. (1605). *Don Juan* in *Oeuvres Complètes*, Vol. 3. Paris: Nelson.

O'Connor, N., and Ryan, J. (1993). *Wild Desires and Mistaken Identities: Lesbianism and Psychoanalysis*. London: Virago, 1993.

Orbach, S. (1986). *Hunger Strike: The Anorectic's Struggle as a Metaphor for Our Age*. New York: Norton.

_____. (2000). *The Impossibility of Sex*. New York: Penguin.

Osherson, S. (1986). *Finding Our Fathers*. New York: Free Press.

Parker, R. (1995). *Mother Love, Mother Hate*. New York: Basic Books.

Peacock, M. (1989). *Take Heart*. New York: Vintage.

Perelman, R. (1999). *Ten to One* (selected poems). Hanover, NH: Wesleyan University Press.

Plato (1953). *Euthyphro, Crito, Apology and Symposium*. South Bend, IN: Regnery/ Gateway.

Poster, M. (1978). *Critical Theory of the Family*. New York: Seabury Press.

Rank, O. (1975). *The Don Juan Legend*, translated by D. Winter. Princeton, NJ: Princeton University Press.

Ray, P. (1989). *Une saison chez Lacan*. Paris: Robert Laffont.

Rich, A. (1976). *Of Woman Born: Motherhood as Experience and Institution*. New York: Norton.

Rudnytsky, P. (1987). *Freud and Oedipus*. New York: Columbia University Press.

_____. (1991). *The Psychoanalytic Vocation: Rank, Winnicott, and the Legacy of Freud*. New Haven: Yale University Press.

Sacks, O. (1987). *The Man Who Mistook His Wife for a Hat*. New York: Harper & Row.

Samuels, A. (1993). *The Political Psyche*. London: Routledge.

_____. (2001). *Politics on the Couch: Citizenship and the Internal Life*. London: Profile Books.

Sayers, J. (1995). *The Man Who Never Was*. New York: Basic Books.

Scharff, D., and Scharff, J.(1987). *Object Relations Family Therapy*. Northvale, NJ: Jason Aronson.

Schneiderman, S. (1980). *Returning to Freud: Clinical Psychoanalysis in the School of Lacan*. New Haven: Yale University Press.

_____. (1983). *Jacques Lacan: The Death of an Intellectual Hero*. Cambridge, MA: Harvard University Press.

Schopenhauer, A. (1819/1969). *The World as Will and Representation*, translated by E. Payne. New York: Dover.

_____. (1851/1974). *Parerga and Paralipomena*. Vol. II. New York: Oxford University Press.

_____. (1851/1988). *Parerga und Paralipomena*. Vol. II. Zurich: Haffmans-Verlag.

_____. (1925). *The Essays of Arthur Schopenhauer*, translated by T. Saunders. New York: Willey Book Co.

Schwartz, J. (1992). *The Creative Moment: How Science Made Itself Alien to Western Culture*. New York: HarperCollins.

_____. (1996). "Physics, philosophy, psychoanalysis and ideology: On engaging with Adolf Grubaum." *Psychoanalytic Dialogues*, *6*, pp. 503–513.

Sennett, R., and Cobb, J. (1972). *The Hidden Injuries of Class*. New York: Knopf.

Sharpe, S. (2000). *The Ways We Love*. New York: Guilford.

Shaw, G. (1903/1977). *Man and Superman*. New York: Penguin.

Silverman, K. (1988). *The Acoustic Mirror: The Female Voice in Psychoanalysis and Cinema*. Bloomington: Indiana University Press.

Simon, C. (1997). *Madhouse: Growing Up in the Shadow of Mentally Ill Siblings*. New York: Penguin.

Sinason, V. (Ed.). (1998). *Memory in Dispute*. London: Karnac Books.

Slater, L. (1996). *Welcome to My Country*. New York: Random House.

Solomon, A. (2001). *Noonday Demon*. New York: Scribner.

Sophocles. (1947). *The Theban Plays*, translated by E. Watling. New York: Penguin.

Spock, B. (1998). *Baby and Child Care*. New York: Pocket Books.

Steinem, G. (1992). *Revolution from Within*. Boston: Little, Brown & Co.

Stringer, L. (1998). *Grand Central Winter*. New York: Seven Stories Press.

Sulloway, F. (1982). "Darwin and his finches: The evolution of a legend." *Journal of the History of Biology*, *15*, pp. 1–53.

Turkle, S. (1978/1992). *Psychoanalytic Politics: Jacques Lacan and Freud's French Revolution*. New York: Guilford.

Vaughan, S. (1997). *The Talking Cure*. New York: Henry Holt.

Walker, A. (1992). *Possessing the Secret of Joy*. New York: Pocket Books.

Weiner, J. (1994). *The Beak of the Finch*. New York: Vintage.

West, C. (1993). *Race Matters*. Boston: Beacon Press.

Winer, R. (1994). *Close Encounters: A Relational View of the Therapeutic Process*. Northvale, NJ: Jason Aronson.

Winnicott, D. (1958/1975). *Through Paediatrics to Psycho-Analysis*. New York: Basic Books.

——————. (1965/1966). *The Maturational Processes and the Facilitating Environment: Studies in the Theory of Emotional Development*. New York: International University Press.

——————. (1971/1984). *Playing and Reality*. London: Tavistock.

——————. (1971/1985). *Therapeutic Consultations in Child Psychiatry*. London: Hogarth Press.

——————. (1977). *The Piggle: An Account of the Psychoanalytic Treatment of a Little Girl*, edited by I. Ramzy. New York: International University Press.

——————. (1989). *Psychoanalytic Explorations*, edited by C. Winnicott, R. Shepherd, and M. Davis. Cambridge, MA: Harvard University Press.

Woolf, V. (1929). *A Room of One's Own*. London: Harcourt, Brace and World.

Wright, E. (1992). *Psychoanalysis and Feminism: A Critical Dictionary*. London: Basil Blackwell.

Young-Bruehl, E. (1996). *The Anatomy of Prejudices*. Cambridge, MA: Harvard University Press.

Zizek, S. (1989). *The Sublime Object of Ideology*. London: Verso.

——————. (2001). *Did Somebody Say "Totalitarianism"?* London: Verso.

ACKNOWLEDGMENTS

I thank my editor, Jo Ann Miller, and my agent, Leslie Daniels, for encouraging me to write a book about psychoanalysis for a general audience.

Thanks to Molly Peacock for graciously giving permission to quote from her poem "There Must Be," which appears in her collection *Take Heart*.

For giving this book and its author tender asylum in New York and London, I thank the Women's Therapy Centre, and especially: Kathlyn Conway, Wendy Miller, Audrey Wolf, Laura Kogel, Lela Zaphiropoulos, Luise Eichenbaum, Anne Leiner, Carol Bloom, and Susie Orbach. They have created an intellectual home in the world for women who run with psychoanalysis and feminism. Also in London: I wish to thank Erica Davies, director of the Freud Museum, for being always generous with her time and expertise during my yearly visits.

Richard Hardack read and criticized every chapter while writing a novel, finishing law school, and making it all seem easy. Much love to him and to others who read early drafts and helped in ways various: Jack Hartke, Annie Steinberg, Nancy Hollander, Sheila Sharpe, Rebecca Barry, Jacqueline Falkenheim, Enid Balint, Dennis Debiak, Jacques Hassoun, Edwin Harari, Chadli Sehili, June Avereyt, Maya Sharma, Gail Kalin, Joe Walsh, Chris Lane, Dale Satorsky, Linda Hopkins, Fred Sander, Carolyn Wulff, and Stewart Moody.

I thank the members of the Philadelphia Lacan study group, which met for five years in my apartment, and especially: Vicki Mahaffey, Patricia Gherovici, and Jean-Michel Rabaté.

I am grateful also to Dr. Paola Mieli, director of *Après Coup* in New York, for her excellent seminars on Lacan and clinical supervision groups.

I thank Bea Kreloff, Edith Isaac-Rose, and Lynne Sharon Schwartz of the Art Workshop International in Assisi, for a wonderful writing course in the summer of 2000.

Much love goes to Fanyi Zeng, who is just a tad smarter than the average professional musician with an M.D. and a Ph.D. from the University of Pennsylvania. Also a computer virtuoso, she orchestrated an operation that saved my ship. *Xie xie, mei-mei!*

Elizabeth Gilbert is a genius, yes, and I was pleased to include many of her suggestions here. However, I simply could not title my "Don Juan" chapter "Touched by a Veterinarian."

The presence of Augie Hermann is like an acre of jasmine in a dot-com world. Writing this book would have been much more difficult without her Virgilian sense of direction.

The person I admire most on the planet is Sister of Mercy Mary Scullion, who, with Joan Dawson, set out in 1989 to solve our city's homelessness problem. I am as honored to be a Project H.O.M.E. volunteer as I was to have had Sister read one of my chapters. Proceeds from this book will go to Project H.O.M.E.

Praise and love to Bernard F. Stehle, *amicus mirabilis*, man of letters, and fabulous dancer, for his delicate acts of literary rescue during the book's final stages.

My deepest gratitude goes to the patients who have allowed me to write about them. May their brilliant act of generosity illuminate the folly of our culture's growing taste for the unexamined life.

Deborah Anna Luepnitz
Philadelphia, July 2001

INDEX

Pregnancy, 3, 31–35, 52, 124–125, 132. *See also* Abortion
Pre-Oedipal stage, 189–190
Privacy, definitions of, 3–4
Projective identification, 29, 94, 129–130, 137, 253
Prozac, 8, 131, 234
Psychosis, 52, 213
Psychosomatic disorders: and back pain, 152, 156, 183, 188
  and diabetes, 66–102
  research on, 80–81
"Publish or perish" system, 153

Race and racism, 96, 125, 152, 162, 164–165, 191–194, 242, 258–259
Rank, Otto, 109, 110, 149
Real, realm of the, 99
Rebellion, in adolescence, 72
Recognition, hunger for, 161–162
Reflection, increasing the capacity for, 62
Religion: Buddhism, 6, 7
  Catholicism, 70
  Hinduism, 7
  Orthodox Judaism, 68–70, 85
Repeat, compulsion to, 132–133
Repression, 3, 237
Resistance, 12–14, 78–79, 154, 193
Roth, Philip, 11

Safety, atmosphere of, 14
Samuels, Andrew, 148
Schopenhauer, Arthur, 2–8. *See also* Porcupine dilemma
Sciatica. *See* back pain
Selective serotonin reuptake inhibitors (SSRIs), 8–9, 131, 235. *See also* Medications
Self: and borderline personalities, 213–214, 229
  and boundaries, 3, 121, 191
  "caretaker," 109
  and dependency, 46, 157, 163
  -esteem, 49
  false, and depression, 109
  and the hunger for recognition, 161–162
  -ishness, 89–92, 155
  and loneliness, 4–5, 106, 151
  -mutilation, 210

-pity, 75
psychology, 161
-reliance, 8, 46, 152
and repression, 3, 237
and resistance, 12–14, 78–79, 193
and the significance of names, 175–177
and the splitting off of painful emotions, 94, 130
true, 109
See also Identification; Personalities
Sennett, Richard, 49
Sentimentality, 109
Sexual abuse, 18–19, 170–171, 224–225, 234, 257
Sexuality: and abstinence, 110–111, 117, 171
  and birth control, 53, 57–58, 61, 63, 131–132
  and castration, 52
  and "Don Juan," 106, 110–111, 115–117, 131, 137–138
  in dreams, 51
  enjoyment of, 61–62
  and heterosexuality, 92, 169, 237–238
  and homosexuality, 113–114, 137, 141, 211, 235–243
  in Lacan, 15–16
  loss of interest in, 106, 115–117, 131, 235
  and pregnancy, 52–53
  and puberty, 92
  and reasons for getting married, 26
  renewed interest in, 181–183
  and the termination of analysis, 169
Sexually-transmitted diseases, 115–116, 131–133, 142–143, 243
Shame, 92
Shoah, 94
Silence: regarding sexual abuse, 224
  during therapy sessions, 62–63, 89, 114–115, 120, 128
Sin-eating (Welsh custom), 233, 245, 260
Sleep disorders, 150, 196
Smoking, 220
Socrates, 5
Solitude, 6, 7, 249
Splitting off, of feelings, 94, 130
Spock, Benjamin, 8, 46
Squiggles, game of, 85–86

ABOUT THE AUTHOR

Deborah Anna Luepnitz, Ph.D., is on the Clinical Faculty of the Department of Psychiatry at the University of Pennsylvania School of Medicine. She is the author of *Child Custody* (1982) and *The Family Interpreted* (1988) and is a contributing author to the *Cambridge Companion to Lacan* (forthcoming). Dr. Luepnitz is a member of the Women's Therapy Centre Institute in New York. She maintains a private practice in Philadelphia.